EUROPEAN SOCIETY FOR MEDICAL ONCOLOGY ANNUAL MEETING IN NICE

Preparation of Abstracts for Direct Reproduction

ENGLISH ABSTRACTS ONLY!

The Abstract texts must begin with a statement of the main purpose of the study. This must be followed by a statement of the methods used.

Precise results to support the conclusions must be presented in an easily comprehensible manner.

The conclusions reached must be precisely stated.

References cannot be included as a part of the abstract.

The typing area is 12.5 x 17.0 cm per abstract. It will be reduced to 65% during reproduction.

Please arrange the text within the outline as follows:

- TITLE in capital letters.
- Continue on the same line with author's names, preceded by initials.
  Do not add Prof., Dr., etc.
- Separate title and author's names from the following text by typing a line
  from left to right across the whole typing area.
- Begin text of abstract on a new line without indentation.
- At the end of the abstract have a blank line, then type full address of
  first author, or institute where the research work was done.

The abstracts will be reproduced directly from the typescript by a photo-graphic process, so there cannot be any subsequent alterations. If a type-script is considered to be unsuitable for reproduction, only the title can be printed. The typist should therefore carefully follow these instructions.

Type the text including any tables in single-line spacing on the special paper provided. Take care not to type outside the outline.

For good reproduction, the typing should be sharp and regular.
Therefore, please:

(1) *Use an electric typewriter.*
(2) *Clean the type before starting.*
(3) *Use a new black ribbon. (This is essential)*
(4) *Set the pressure at the maximum.*
(5) *Symbols (not on the typewriter) should be inserted in Indian ink with a fine pen or black ball-point pen.*
(6) *Do not use other colours — they will not print.*
(7) *Avoid erasures and smudges. Use white correcting fluid (Tipp-ex) or white patches to insert corrections.*
(8) *Two sheets of special paper are enclosed in case the first attempt is a failure.*

The original of the abstract must reach the Congress Office on the date stated in the invitation at the latest. Manuscripts received after this date cannot be included.

Offprints will not be supplied.

European Society for
Medical Oncology

Abstracts
of the 6th Annual Meeting

Nice, December 6–8, 1980

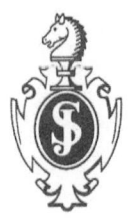 Springer-Verlag Berlin Heidelberg GmbH

ISBN 978-3-662-39221-8   ISBN 978-3-662-40234-4 (eBook)
DOI 10.1007/978-3-662-40234-4

1

IS TOXICITY CORRELATED WITH EFFICACY IN MULTIPLE DRUG CHEMOTHERAPY FOR ADVANCED PRIMARY LUNG CANCER? A. Aapro, M. Forni, P. Sappino, M. Berchtold, P. Alberto

392 patients with advanced primary lung cancer were treated with 5 regimens of chemotherapy including Cyclophosphamide, Methotrexate, Vincristine, Procarbazine, Hydroxyurea, Adriamycin and CCNU.
The responses of more than 50% were registered after 8 weeks of treatment. During this same period, the intensity of leucopenia, thrombocytopenia, vomiting, other digestive toxicity, neurologic disorders and alopecia were graded according to the worst observation from 0 to 4.
The results show that there is no correlation between the grade of toxicity and the rate of respons either for the entire group or for subgroups of patients as defined by cell type, degree of dissemination, age or performance status.
These results show that the search for maximum toxicity does not warrant the best possible response to chemotherapy in primary lung cancer.

Division of Oncology, Hospital Cantonal
1211 Geneva 4, Switzerland

2

PHASE I TRIAL WITH CARMINOMYCIN (CMM). R. Abele, M. Rozencweig, J.J. Body, S.D. Reich, L. Lenaz, S.T.Crooke and Y. Kenis.

CMM is a new anthracycline derivative that was reported to induce lesser cardiotoxicity than Adriamycin (ADM) in experimental systems. In this phase I study, the drug was given by rapid iv injection repeated every 3 to 4 wks in adult patients with advanced solid tumors, mainly lung or head and neck cancer. None of the patients had prior anthracycline treatment, abnormal cardiac function, bilirubine $\geq$ 1.5 mg% or creatinine $\geq$ 1.5 mg%. Median age was 63 yrs and median performance status (PS) was 70. The trial was initiated at a starting dose of 12 mg/m2 and dose levels were escalated up to 22 mg/m2. A total of 35 courses were administered to 19 patients. Only 2 patients received more than 2 courses. Leucopenia was dose-limiting and dose dependent with a steep dose-response relationship. Median WBC nadir was > 4000 at 15 mg/m2 and 1100 at 22 mg/m2. It occurred on median day 12 with generally prompt recovery. Leucopenia appeared to vary widely within each dose level. Thrombocytopenia (<100,000) was seen in 3 courses. Myelosuppression was noticeably more severe in patients with low PS a/o massive liver invasion. Nonhematological toxic effects were negligible and included minor to moderate alopecia in 8 patients, minimal nausea in 4 courses, transient electrocardiographic changes consisting of ST-T wave modifications in 2 courses, and fever in 1 course. Phlebitis without sloughing at the injection site was seen in 1 patient. Drug-induced congestive heart failure was not observed. No objective antitumor effect could be documented. CMM is more potent than ADM. At doses achieving similar leucopenia, other toxic effects are much less pronounced with CMM. Conclusions on the relative cardiotoxicity of CMM must await additional trials with more prolonged treatments. A dose-schedule of 20 mg/m2 q 3 wks may be recommended for phase II studies with CMM in good risk outpatients.

Inst.Jules Bordet, Brussels, Belgium, Univ.Mass.Worcester, Ma, Bristol-Myers,New York,NY, Bristol Lab.,Syracuse, NY.

3

A PHASE II STUDY OF COMBINED CIS-PLATINUM AND BLEOMYCIN GIVEN OVER A 5/6 DAY PERIOD IN 83 PATIENTS WITH MEASURABLE SQUAMOUS CELL CARCINOMAS. J. Aguilera[1], L. Israel[1], J.L. Breau[1], J. Soudant[1], J.C. Penot[2], P. Grateau[3], L. Soubeyrand[4]

Cis-platinum was given at 20 mg/m2/day in 3 hours following hydration and mannitol. Bleomycin was given simultaneously at 6 mg/m2/day in continuous infusion, 5 consecutive days in preoperative patients and 6 consecutive days in non-operable patients, for 2 to 3 courses, one every 3 weeks. Ancillary treatment consisted of prednisone, magnesium chloride and calcium gluconate. Were treated: operable head and neck ca: 32; unresectable head and neck patients not previously irradiated: 6, unresectable head and neck patients with recurrence after irradiation: 11; squamous cell ca of the lung: 13; unresectable oesophageal ca: 10 (2 recurrences after irradiation); cervix ca: 2 operable cases, 3 with pelvic recurrence (1 after irradiation); miscellaneous: 5 disseminated cases (2 testicular, 1 breast, 1 bladder, 1 ano-rectal). Toxicity consisted of 3 pulmonary fibrosis, reversible at the 2nd and 3rd course in patients receiving a 6 day course. No renal toxicity or hematologic toxicity was seen. Response rates were: operable head and neck: 23/32 >50% responses (71%) (6 CR); inoperable unirradiated head and neck: 5/6 >50% (2 CR); inoperable irradiated head and neck: 5/11 (no CR); bronchial ca: 10/13 (3 CR histological); oesophageal: 6/10 > 50% (2 CR histological); cervix: 3/5 PR (1 CR); miscellaneous: 5/5 (1 CR in breast). Duration of response is not available due to immediate secondary therapy local and/or systemic. This regime shows very high response rates in previously poorly responding sites, and is superior to cis-platinum and Bleomycin in 1 day courses. Due to cumulative toxicity of Bleomycin, it should be employed mainly in preoperative or pre-irradiation cases.

[1]CHU Avicenne, 93000 Bobigny. [2]CHU Orléans, 45000 Orléans. [3]Hôpital Militaire du Val de Grâce, 75005 Paris. [4]Hôpital Militaire Bégin, 94160 St. Mandé

4

AN EORTC PHASE II TRIAL OF THIOPROLINE (NORGAMEM, NSC 25-855) IN PATIENTS WITH ADVANCED SQUAMOUS CELL CARCINOMA OF THE HEAD AND NECK (HN). P. Alberto, A. Brugarolas, H.H. Hansen, F. Cavalli, A. Clarysse, W. Gallmeir, H. Hørst, K. James, R. Pinedo (for the EORTC Early Clinical Trials Cooperative Group)

Thioproline (TP) (Thiazolidine-4-carboxylic acid) is a chelating agent of low molecular weight releasing free SH-radicals in vivo. Recently, Gosalvez et al. suggested that TP could restore contact inhibition in malignant cell cultures and reverse the lack of cell differentiation. It was speculated that TP could modify tumor cells by reverse transformation into non-malignant cells. TP is inactive in experimental tumor systems.
TP (5 to 40 mg/kg daily IV or IM) was used by Brugarolas in a Phase I-II trial in patients with various tumors, predominantly squamous cell carcinoma of the HN. The data reported are suggestive of high activity. However, in another preliminary Phase II trial of TP (20 mg/kg daily x 5 continuous IV infusion) Alberto et al. observed one short term response in 7 patients with HN tumors (proc. ASCO 1980).
An EORTC Phase II trial of TP was initiated in February 1980 in patients with squamous cell carcinoma of the HN or of the lung. All patients must have measurable tumor lesions not amenable to surgery or radiation therapy and a Karnofsky index of 50 or more. TP dose is 40 mg/kg daily divided in 4 IM injections (q6H) for 6 weeks or more. 13 patients out of 20 are provisorily evaluable with one partial response. The only observed toxicity is a transient mental confusion or aggressiveness in a few patients. The study continues. A larger number of patients is needed for a final assessment.

Division of Oncology, Hôpital Cantonal
1211 Geneva 4, Switzerland

5

ADJUVANT THERAPY WITH INTERFERON OF A LIMB OSTEOSARCOMA INDUCED BY RADIOACTIVE CERIUM IN THE RAT.

M. Allouche[1], C. Jasmin[1], J.G. Judde[1], H. Delbruck[1], C. Fizames[1], M.Morin[2] and J. Lafuma[2].

The osteosarcoma induced by injection of radioactive Cerium chloride into the hind leg of Sprague Dawley rats shares many similarities with its human counterpart. The tumor shows the typical histology of human osteosarcoma, a low mean labelling index after a pulse labeling with tritiated thymidine and metastases mainly in the lungs. Futhermore, we have shown that lung metastases are present in the lungs of 50% to 70% of animals at the time of detection of the primary tumor.

A pilot trial conducted by Strander et al. has shown that treatment with interferon could delay or even prevent the development of lung metastases which are also present in human patients at the time of diagnosis. However, the rarity of the tumor and the paucity of human interferon has not yet allowed confirmatory trials.

We have conducted a randomized trial of adjuvant therapy with rat interferon in rats bearing tumors induced by radioactive cerium. As soon as a tumor was palpated, the tumor was removed by amputation and the animal received ip injection of 0.25 ml of PBS or 8×10^5 units of semi-purified rat cell culture interferon. Animals were treated 3 times per week. Treatment was continued up to a maximum of 2 months. No difference was found between the two groups according to the percentage of lung metastases, their mean number, the size and the mean survival time. This trial using a protocol very similar to the human trial shows the interest of induced osteosarcomas to perform experimental trials of adjuvant therapy in a rare human tumor. However different schedules with higher doses of interferon must be used before concluding that interferon is without efficacy in the experimental rat osteosarcoma.

AcknowledgementD.G.R.S.T. projet 278/B
1. I.C.I.G. Hopital Paul Brousse Villejuif (France)
2. C.E.A. Department de Radiotoxicologie Fontenay-aux-Roses (France)

6

A PHASE I TRIAL AND PHARMACOKINETICS IN BABOON OF A NEW PLATINUM ANTITUMOR COMPOUND, PHIC. J.P. Armand and J.P. Macquet

PHIC is a new platinum antitumor compound with a higher water solubility (> 1500 mg/ml), lower toxicity (LDo = 150 mg/kg) and better antitumoral activity (TI = 25 in L1210 and 17.5 in S180) than cisplatin (2 mg/ml, LDo = 9 mg/kg, TI = 6.5 in L1210 and 6 in S180).

Escalating doses of 100, 150, or 200 mg/kg were injected (daily x 1 i.v. every 21 days) in baboon by a 10 minute infusion during short anesthesia.

The 100 mg/kg treatment was given 6 times, once every three weeks. Creatinine levels and blood parameters were found unchanged; only a slight decrease could be detected in hemostasis values, vomiting was very mild and change in body weight was less than 10 %.

For the 150 mg/kg schedule, 2 limiting toxicities appeared: nephrotoxicity (creatinine increased on days 5 to 10) which was the cause of death and myelotoxicity which was maximum on day 11.

In the 200 mg/kg schedule, nephrotoxicity and myelotoxicity were decreased by prehydration. However, coagulation disorders appeared immediately after injection and disappeared over 10 days. They consist of a decrease in plasma prothrombin time from 100 to 10 % with proconvertin VII < 5 % and prothrombin II < 30 %. This decrease is not due to a diffuse intravascular coagulation and has no clinical expression.

Using atomic absorption spectrophotometry (detection limit of 50 pg Pt) pharmacokinetics of PHIC was measured in total blood, after a 100 mg/kg injection during 1 minute without hydration. The results (µM Pt) are :

1mn	2mn	3mn	4mn	5mn	10mn	30mn	1h	5h	24h	48h	72h
1047	749	650	601	542	315	153	97.8	49.2	31.6	17.2	12.3

Centre Claudius Regaud, 11 rue Piquemil, 31052 TOULOUSE CEDEX, France.

7

RADIOLOGY AS A PROGNOSTIC FACTOR FOR 30 PATIENTS WITH OSTEOGENIC SARCOMA. J.P. Armand, A. Pons, J. Douchez, M. Carton, P.F. Combes

Iatrogenic risks often observed with adjuvant treatment of osteogenic sarcoma led us to search for a prognostic factor which would allow better selection of a high risk group.

30 patients treated from 1967 to 1978 at the Centre Claudius Regaud have been analyzed. All were verified by surgical biopsy. Were considered as cured all patients who never developed metastases and showed no evidence of disease (NED) at least 30 months after treatment of the tumor.

9 patients were cured at 30 and 44 months and at 5,6,7,7, 8, 9 and 11 years. The radiological study was carried out using frontal and profile X-rays; there were 4 types of patterns based solely on the descriptive picture in the light of Lodwick's work:

I   : geographical patterns (clear edges)
II : moth-eaten patterns (several small confluent groups)
III : permeated pattern (confluent tiny gaps)
IV : homogeneous condensation

According to the relative participation of lysis and condensation, we compared series A (I+II) and series B (III + IV) to the survival rate: 9/18 patients were cured in series A, none of 12 survived in series B. Comparision is significant at 1% (p <0.01). Series A was not priveleged over B regarding adjuvant therapy (7A vs 4B) or topographical distribution (femur, humerus 11A vs 7B; tibia, distal bones 7A vs 5B).

Tomodensitometry should allow more accurate definition of what already seems a good prognostic criterion.

Centre Claudius Regaud, 11 rue Piquemil
31052 Toulouse, France

8

PHARMACOKINETICS OF VP 16-213 USING A NEW HPLC ASSAY
A M Arnold , M Dodson, A Renwick and J M A Whitehouse

To date no simple assay has been available to directly measure plasma levels of the podophyllotoxin derivative VP 16-213. We propose an assay, utilising High-Pressure Liquid Chromatograpy, to investigate the pharmacokinetics of this drug. The VP 16-213 peak is clearly identifiable and height of the peak is an accurate parameter for measuring VP 16-213 in blood (correlation = 0.9789). The extraction process recovers 72-87% of the drug from plasma with a reproducibility of within $\pm$ 2%. Drugs commonly used together with VP 16-213 do not interfere with the VP 16-213 peak. The drug is stable in plasma for at least 22 weeks, and in normal saline at therapeutic concentration is stable for at least 20 hours. Haemolysis of a blood sample does not affect the concentration of the drug in the plasma and contrary to expectation the drug does not appear to deteriorate when exposed to light.

Six   patients were given a 30 minute infusion of VP 16-213 in saline at a dose of 200 mg/m^2. VP 16-213 plasma decay kinetics appear to follow a triexponential function and correspond to a three-compartment open model (mammillary type). Mean values for the parameters are: P=20.55µg/ml; A=19.98µg/ml; B=1.29µg/ml; π =2.12hr^{-1}; α=0.16hr^{-1} ; β =0.029 hr^{-1}. Plasma clearance was 47.10 ml/min, and renal clearance 13.56 ml/min. The half-life of the terminal elimination phase was 43.22 hours. Bioavailability studies comparing plasma concentrations of intravenous versus oral administration of VP 16-213 are ongoing but provisional data suggests that the bioavailability of the gelatin capsule is approximately 50%.

CRC Medical Oncology Unit, University of Southampton, Southampton, England.

9

INTERACTION OF VP 16-213 WITH DNA REPAIR ANTAGONISTS.
A.M.Arnold, J.M.Whitehouse.

The podophyllotoxin derivative VP 16-213 can apparently
cause single stranded breaks in D.N.A. capable of repair.
Several compounds are known to be powerful inhibitors of
D.N.A. repair so it was of interest to study the interactions of VP 16-213 with chloroquine and caffeine. Female
D.B.A. mice weighing 20 gms were inoculated subcutaneously
with 1×10^5 TLX lymphoma cells. Three days after inocu-
lation the animals were treated with VP 16-213, together
with either chloroquine (20-40 mg/kg) by i.p. injection
or caffeine 0.125-1% added to the drinking water. By way
of a control Vincristine, a drug not thought to damage
D.N.A., was also tested with chloroquine. Results were
expressed as increased lifespan (ILS) over untreated controls. VP 16-213 alone (6.25 mg/kg and 12.5 mg/kg) produced an ILS of 9% and 30% respectively. VP 16-213 in the
same doses but together with 40 mg/kg chloroquine produced ILS of 78% and 76% respectively (P = 0.05). By contrast
chloroquine did not enhance the effect of Vincristine.
1% caffeine added to drinking water of animals given VP
16-213 produced a significant but less marked ILS. These
preliminary observations provide further evidence that
the mode of action of VP 16-213 may be due to the formation of single stranded breaks in D.N.A. although it is
possible that other mechanisms may be responsible for the
apparent synergism.

CRC Medical Oncology Unit, University of Southampton,
Southampton, England.

11

GAS-LIQUID CHROMATOGRAPHY (G.L.C.) ASSAY FOR 1,3,5-
TRIGLYCIDYL-S-TRIAZINETRIONE (αTGT). G. Atassi[+], A. Menil[++];
P. Dumont[+], C. Dorlet[++] and G. Lagrange[++].

αTGT has shown very high antitumor activity against
various murine solid tumors and leukemias and entered
phase I clinical trials. With a view to prepare for
pharmacokinetic and protein-binding studies in man, we
have performed a G.L.C. assay using a glass column
conditioned by a stationary phase (2 % OV-17 on chromosorb
W-HP 100/200 mesh) and a thermo-ionic detector.
αTGT-enriched human plasma was extracted by chloroform
during 20 min. at room temperature. Organic phase was
evaporated, then resuspended in chloroform and injected.
The assay was performed as follows: the column was heated
at 300°C under helium flux (30 ml/min.) during 12 h.
(Oven temp.: 245°C; injection temp.: 265°C; volume of the
injected sample: 1 μl). Retention time of αTGT was 2 min.
and that of internal standard (caffein) 0.59 min. The
results showed that the amount recovered is directly pro-
portional to the initial concentration and reaches
values of 97 % after 20 min. extraction. The linearity of
the assay permits the use of caffein as internal standard.
Using this assay in a preliminary pharmacokinetic study
in mice indicated a rapid plasmatic clearance after a
single intravenous injection of 180 mg/kg of αTGT (the
half-lives of the two decay phases are 4 sec. and 96 sec.
respectively). The reproducibility of this assay
demonstrates it is useful for pharmacological studies and
for understanding the effect of αTGT in man and in animals.

[+] Institut Jules Bordet, Service de Médecine et d'Investigation clinique, Rue Héger-Bordet 1, 1000 Bruxelles,
Belgique

[++] Université Libre de Bruxelles, Institut de Pharmacie, Laboratoire de Chimie pharmaceutique organique, Bruxelles,
Belgique

10

1,3,5-TRIGLYCIDYL-S-TRIAZINETRIONE (αTGT). A NEW ANTI-
TUMOR AGENT. G. Atassi, P. Dumont and D. Gangjî.

The antitumor properties of the α and β stereoisomers of
1,3,5-triglycidyl-s-triazinetrione (TGT) were investigated
on various transplantable murine tumors. Although the two
stereoisomers showed high therapeutic activity against
P388 and L1210 leukemias when administered intraperitoneal-
ly (i.p.), αTGT, a more water-soluble compound, was
superior to the β form in increasing lifespan (I.L.S.) of
treated animals and in inducing (at 50 mg/kg X 9)
long-term survivals of treated animals (70 % over 90 days).
αTGT demonstrated antitumor effect against advanced L1210
leukemia (I.L.S. of 119 % at 50 mg/kg X 9) and was still
very active when administered orally or intravenously. Its
activity against intracerebral L1210 and ependymoblastoma
was moderate and yet significant (I.L.S. of 51 and 65 %
respectively). This suggests that αTGT may cross, at least
partially, the meningeal barrier. I.p. treatment with αTGT
significantly inhibited tumor growth and lung metastases
of Lewis lung carcinoma and tumor growth of colon adenocarcinoma 38 and induced 60 to 100 % cures in mice bearing
i.p. colon adenocarcinoma 26. An agar clonogenic assay was
performed using human mammary cell line Evsa-T. 10 μg/ml
per 1 h. incubation inhibited the colony formation by 60 %.
Doses between 1-0.01 μg/ml did not produce significant
colony inhibition. Finally, the high in vivo activity of
αTGT on normal P388 tumor and on a subline of the latter
which is markedly resistant to cyclophosphamide (I.L.S. of
378 % plus 30 % cures at 40 mg/kg X 9) warrants further
study with this agent.

Institut Jules Bordet, Service de Médecine et d'Investigation clinique, Rue Héger-Bordet 1, 1000-Bruxelles, Belgique.

12

GLYCOSYLTRANSFERASE ACTIVITIES OF NEOPLASTIC HE-
MATOPOETIC CELLS - MARKERS FOR CELL MATURATION?
Augener,W. and G.Brittinger

Neoplastic transformation of cells may be accompanied by alterations of the composition and metabolism of cellular glycoconjugates. Therefore,
the study of glycosyltransferase activities, responsible for the assembly of complex carbohy-
drates, may contribute to elucidate the enigma
of neoplastic cells. The activities of fucosyl-
transferase (Fuc-T) and N-Acetylneuraminyltrans-
ferase (NeuAc-T) were determined in lysates of
various leukemic cells arrested at different
stages of maturation and of normal T- and B-lymphocytes. Isolated cells were characterized by
surface markers. Fuc-T and NeuAc-T activities
were quantitated by the transfer of 14C-Fuc and
14C-NeuAc to exogenous acceptors from sugar nucleotides. Leukemic non-T/non-B lymphoblasts and
myeloblasts arrested at an early stage of maturation displayed high Fuc-T and low NeuAc-T activities. Leukemic T-lymphoblasts, further developed
along the T-lymphocyte lineage, showed increased
NeuAc-T activity. In contrast, neoplastic B-cells
revealed low Fuc-T and either low or high levels
of NeuAc-T activity. Normal T- and B-lymphocytes
showed low activities of both enzyme systems.
These data suggest that during the process of
cell maturation the expression of Fuc-T precedes
that of NeuAc-T. Neoplastic cells from cancer
patients have been implicated as a source of
plasma glycosyltransferases. The reported increased levels of either Fuc-T or NeuAc-T activities
in the plasma of cancer patients may be related
to the specific states of maturation at which
the individual neoplastic cells are arrested.

Div. of Hematology, Dept. of Medicine, Universi-
tätsklinikum Essen, Essen, FRG. // SFB 102 , B6

4

13

HUMAN PHARMACOLOGY AND TOXICOLOGY OF 13-CIS-RETINOIC ACID
Pierre Band, Jean-Guy Besner, Robert Leclaire, Geneviève
Diorio, and Mario Beretta Picoli.

Vitamin A and its synthetic analogs (retinoids) inhibit the
development of carcinogen induced pre-neoplastic and neoplastic lesions in a variety of experimental in vitro and
in vivo systems. We report the results of a phase I
pharmacologic and toxicologic study in cancer patients of
the retinoid 13-cis-retinoic acid (13-cis-RA) initiated
prior to evaluating the chemopreventive effect of the
drug in patients having severe dysplasias. A three month
course of daily oral doses of $20mg/m^2$, $35mg/m^2$, $60mg/m^2$,
$90mg/m^2$ and $120mg/m^2$ of 13-cis-RA was given to 2, 6, 6, 1
and 1 patients respectively.

Peak serum concentrations occured at 1 hour after drug
administration, and serum half-life was 16 hours.

Mild dryness of the lips, cheilitis, conjunctivitis and
skin xerosis were seen at all dose levels. Moderate
toxicity consisting of erythemato-squamous skin lesions
and/or serum alkaline phosphatase elevation were observed
in 5 patients treated with $60mg/m^2$ of the drug. Severe
toxicity including headaches, exfoliative dermatitis,
urethritis, and photophobia occurred at doses of $90mg/m^2$
and $120mg/m^2$.

An initial dose of $60mg/m^2$ of 13-cis-RA is suggested for
clinical trials.

(Supported in part by Hoffman LaRoche Ltd., Canada.)

Institut du Cancer de Montréal, 1560 est Sherbrooke,
Montréal Québec, H21 4M1 Canada.

14

EFFECTIVENESS OF COMBINATION CHEMOTHERAPY USING α-DI-
FLUOROMETHYLORNITHINE AND ADRIAMYCIN OR VINDESINE IN THE
TREATMENT OF DIFFERENT ANIMAL TUMORS. J. Bartholeyns

α-Difluoromethylornithine (DFMO, RMI 71.782), a specific,
irreversible inhibitor of ornithine decarboxylase, has
been shown to have antitumoral properties (Prakash et al.
Cancer Res. 38:3059-3062, 1978, Life Sci. 26:181-194,
1980). The effects of DFMO in combination therapy with
Vindesine or Adriamycin have now been investigated in 3
animal models.
1. - Treatment with DFMO, 2 % in drinking water (2.4 g/kg/
day), or with 0.1 mg/kg/week vindesine, i.p., or with 2.5
mg/kg/week adriamycin, i.p., starting 1 day after inocu-
lation of BD2F mice with L1210 cells, increased the mean
survival by 1.2, 1.4 and 2.3 fold respectively. Combination therapy with DFMO resulted in a doubling of survival
in the case of vindesine and in a 3.5 fold increase in
the case of adriamycin with 30 % long term survivors.
2. - Treatment of Buffalo rats with DFMO, 2 % in drinking
water (1.5 g/kg/day), or with 0.2 mg/kg/week vindesine,
i.p., or with 2.5 mg/kg/week adriamycin, i.p., inhibited
the growth of solid intramuscular tumors induced by hepa-
toma tissue culture cells by 60 to 70 % after 2 weeks of
treatment. When the same doses of vindesine or adriamycin
were administered in combination with DFMO the growth of
the tumor was blocked.
3. - Combined treatment of BALBC mice bearing EMT6 sub-
cutaneous solid tumors with DFMO and adriamycin or vindesine resulted in enhanced inhibition of tumor growth compared to single drug therapy. These data indicate that
DFMO combined with vindesine or adriamycin could be an
effective approach to the treatment of various cancers.

Centre de Recherche Merrell International
16, rue d'Ankara
67084 STRASBOURG
FRANCE

15

PILOT STUDIES FOR CARCINOMAS OF THE DIGESTIVE TRACT.
D. Belpomme , C. Gisselbrecht , L. Mignot , M. Marty ,
M. Boiron

85 advanced colorectal carcinomas were treated by three
different chemotherapy regimens. In 40 patients a cyclic
combination (ECR 1) was used consisting of VM 26 60mg/sqm
d. 1, Mitomycin C 12mg/sqm d. 2, CCNU 60mg/sqm d. 3, 4
and 5 FU 400mg/sqm d. 2 to 5. The response rate was 25%
using new nitrosourea derivatives.27 patients were treated with 5 FU 300mg/sqm for 5 days and Chlorozotocin
80mg/sqm d. 1, and 18 additional advanced colorectal cancers with 5 FU 600mg/sqm on weeks 1, 2, 5, 6, 9, Cyclophosphamide 600mg/sqm on weeks 1, 5, 9, Mitomycin C 6mg/
sqm on weeks 1, 9 and RFCNU 300mg/sqm every five weeks.
The response rate was respectively 18% and 16%. None of
the combinations used gave better results than 5 FU alone.
20 advanced gastric carcinomas were treated by the same
cyclic combination (ECR 1). The response rate was 32%
with a median survival for responders of 7.8. months. In
order to improve the results obtained in 61 patients with
the FAM protocol (MacDonald et al.) which gives a 43% partial remission rate, and a median survival of 14 months
for responders, we ran two studies adding to FAM either
chlorozotocin 80mg/sqm or RFCNU 300mg/sqm. The response
rate was 40% in a group of 10 patients treated with FAM-
Chlorozotocin and 28% in 14 patients who had received FAM
RFCNU. The addition of nitrosoureas did not seem to improve the overall result of the FAM combination.
15 patients with advanced esophagus carcinoma were treated by CDDP combination including in 9 patients 5 FU and
Adriamycin and in 6 other patients Bleomycin, Vinblastine. Response rate was 50% with 3 complete remissions. Our
study compares very favorably with the 40% response rate
reported with CDDP alone.
Supported by French-American agrement.

Hôpital Saint Louis, Paris

16

BRONCHUS SMALL CELL ANAPLASTIC CARCINOMA : TREATMENT OF
EXTENSIVE DISEASE BY ADRIAMYCIN , VINCRISTINE, METHO-
TREXATE, CYCLOPHOSPHAMIDE AND RADIOTHERAPY, D. Belpomme,
E. Pujade-Lauraine, C.Gisselbrecht, L. Mignot, M.Grandjean
P. Bouffette, A. Bohu, M. Marty and M. Boiron.

25 patients (mean age 56.3, sex ratio F:M, 7:18) with
advanced bronchus small cell anaplastic carcinoma have
been treated by sequential chemoradiotherapy consisting
of 4 to 6 monthly cycles of AVMC inductive chemotherapy
followed by complementary radiotherapy and M.C. maintenance chemotherapy. AVMC consisted on day 1 of ADRIAMY-
CIN 50 mg./m2 and VINCRISTINE 2 mg./m2, on days 2, 3,
4 and 5 of CYCLOPHOSPHAMIDE IM, 400 mg./m2 per day and
on days 2 and 3 of METHOTREXATE IM 15 mg./m2, 3 times
per day. Complementary radiotherapy was delivered to all
local residual tumors and systematically to the mediastinum, supraclavicular area (35-45 gr.) and CNS up to C_2
(24 gr.). IM chemotherapy maintenance consisted of monthly courses on days 1 and 2 of METHOTREXATE 30 mg./m2 per
day and on days 1, 2 and 3 of CYCLOPHOSPHAMIDE 400 mg/m2
per day.
Based on 20 evaluable patients, overall and complete (CR)
response rates were 90 % (17/20) and 25 % (5/20) respectively ; median survival was 15 months ; there were no
surviving patients at 24 months. Tolerance of chemotherapy was acceptable in all ambulatory patients. Although
encouraging, these results stress nonetheless that chemoradiotherapy should consist of new more intensive therapeutic regimens aimed at increasing CR rates.

Département de Cancérologie. Hôpital Saint-Louis. Paris
(France).

17

ANAMNESTIC COMPARATIVE SELF-APPRAISAL (ACSA) TO MEASURE SUBJECTIVE QUALITY OF LIFE OF CANCER PATIENTS : RESULTS OF A PILOT STUDY. J.Bernheim, M.Buyse

According to a recent literature survey on the quality of life of cancer patients (QL), all measured variables were somatic, functional or otherwise observer-chosen. No measure of subjective QL has thus far been widely applied. With ACSA, the patients score their present level of well-being on a scale ranging between +5, representing their well-being during life's "best" or "happiest" periods and -5, the "worst" or "unhappiest" circumstances. This represents a comprehensive scale of subjective QL. Then sequential estimates of QL are obtained during the course of early symptoms, hospitalization, treatment and follow-up. These scores can be integrated over time, generating "average values" of QL during various phases of disease and treatment. The difference between these averages and remembered QL before disease (ΔACSA) is a measure of impact of disease on a patient's overall well-being. Data on 65 patients with various neoplasms were available for statistical analysis. The impact of disease and treatment on overall well-being as measured by ΔACSA is only loosely correlated with changes in Karnofsky's Performance Status (correlation coefficient, r = .47) and weight changes (r = .31). Statistically significant correlations are associated with life expectancy (P = .004), aggressivity of chemotherapeutic treatment (P = .003), objective response to treatment (P = .04) and other clinically measurable parameters. ACSA is well tolerated, easy to obtain by the somatic therapist and appears reproducible, as evidenced by the preliminary results of a validation study conducted by psychiatrists independent of the somatic therapist. Its psychotherapeutic value and usefulness as a variable expressing results of cancer treatment are under further investigation.

Institut Jules Bordet and E.O.R.T.C. Data Center,
1 rue Héger-Bordet, 1000 Brussels, Belgium.

18

BCG-CWP THERAPY IN HEAD AND NECK CANCER. J. Bier, H.Pickartz, S. Schlesinger, S. Kleinschuster, B. Zbar, H. Rapp, T. Borsos, M. Röllinghoff, H. Wagner.

Experimental studies in guinea pigs have demonstrated successful intratumoral therapy to the primary lesion as well as for the regional metastatic lymph nodes with BCG-CWP (cell-wall-preparation). Tumor regression under this type of therapy was also seen in cows with naturally occuring ocular squamous cell carcinoma. Based on these results the first clinical study for this type of therapy was developed. Patients with head and neck carcinoma stage $T_{1/2}N_0_2M_0$ were randomised. One group was treated only surgically, a second group received preoperative intralesional BCG-CWP. Until now 16 patients were included in each group. After 40 months the CCR (complete cancer remission) in the operative group was 0.45 and in the preoperative BCG-CWP group 0.77 (p=0.075). The cumulative proportion of surviving patients was 0.58 in the operative and 0.72 in the BCG-CWP group (p=0.26). BCG-CWP injection was followed by an increase in body temperature and decrease in peripheral blood lymphocytes. No changes in liver, kidney or other organ function could be observed after BCG-CWP therapy. Complications and severe secondary effects as described for living BCG could not be observed. The histology showed no changes in cell quality before and after injection of BCG-CWP. However, BCG-CWP mediated a significant intra- and peritumoral increase of lymphocytes and histiocytes and the formation of granulomas around the tumor and in the draining lymph nodes. Significant immunological changes as delayed type hypersensitivity and lymphocyte reactivity in vitro could not be detected until now. So far a single preoperative intralesional injection of BCG-CWP is better than radical surgery alone.

Priv. Doz. Dr. Dr. Jürgen Bier, Abteilung für Kiefer- und Plastische Gesichtschirurgie, Klinikum Steglitz, Hindenburgdamm 30, 1000 Berlin 45, West-Germany.

19

COMPUTER ANALYSIS IN THE INVESTIGATION OF MALIGNANT LIVER NEOPLASMS - REPORT OF A CURRENT CLINICAL ULTRASOUND STUDY. H. Bihl, M.L. Sautter, D. Schlaps, M. Kleckow, G.van Kaick, W.J. Lorenz

The principal aim of the work is to give a contribution on accurate tumor staging especially in cases where diffuse echo-alterations make the diagnosis of metastatic infiltration difficult for conventional grey-scale ultrasound as well as for CT, i.e. when definable circumscribed masses are missing.

As previously shown (W.J.Lorenz et al., 1980) computer assisted analysis - meaning the digital recording of A-Scan signals from the parenchyma, signal processing and extracting a number of complex parameters characterizing those signals - turned out to be powerful in differentiating tissue structures.

This communication presents our experience in using the above method for the diagnosis of liver metastasis. So far we examined 36 patients with a histologically confirmed neoplastic alteration of the liver. In 34 cases (about 95% sensitivity) the diagnosis based on the above method was correct, the two false negatives were classified as non malignant alterations or normal parenchyma.

Reference:
W.J. Lorenz et al.: B-Scan kontrollierte A-Scan Computeranalyse bei Leber- und Nierenerkrankungen. In: M. Hinselmann et al. (Ed.): Ultraschalldiagnostik in der Medizin. Thieme 1980

H. Bihl, Institute of Nuclear Medicine, German Cancer Research Center, Heidelberg, Im Neuenheimer Feld 280, D-6900 Heidelberg 1

20

ADRIAMYCIN, BLEOMYCIN, VINBLASTINE & DTIC (ABVD) AS THIRD AND FIRST LINE CHEMOTHERAPY IN ADVANCED BREAST CARCINOMA. S. Biran, E. Gez, J. Yahalom and A. Sulkes

Twenty evaluable patients (pts) with advanced breast carcinoma who had failed prior chemotherapy with Cyclophosphamide, Methotrexate and 5-FU (CMF) and CMF plus Vincristine and prednisone (CMFVP) were given ABVD as third line chemotherapy as follows: A 25 mg/m2, B 15 mg, V 6 mg/m2, and D 300 mg/m2, all IV on days 1 and 14 of each course, every 4 weeks. There were no complete responses. 3 pts (15%) had a partial response (PR), 2 pts (10%) improved (I) less than PR, 3 pts (15%) had stabilization and 12 pts (60%) progressed on this scheme. Median survival from ABVD for responders (PR + I) was 8.5 months and only 4.5 months for progressors. With evidence of activity in heavily pretreated pts with far advanced disease, ABVD was then compared with CMFVP as first line chemotherapy in metastatic breast carcinoma. Nineteen pts have been entered into this randomized, on-going study. About half of the pts in each arm have shown an objective response; median duration of CR + PR with CMFVP is at present 13+ months and 8+ months for ABVD. Although both regimens appear equally effective as first line chemotherapy in breast carcinoma, ABVD seems to be less well tolerated.

Department of Radiation and Clinical Oncology
Hebrew University - Hadassah Medical School
Jerusalem, Israel

21

PHASE I EVALUATION OF THE COMBINATION METHOTREXATE-MITO-
MYCIN C. J.J. Body, M. Rozencweig and Y. Kenis

Synergistic antitumor activity was recently reported in
murine leukemias with combinations of methotrexate (MTX)
and mitomycin C (MMC) (Mabel AACR 21, 291, 1980). We initiated a pilot study using MMC on d1 and MTX on d1 and 8
in head and neck cancer. Drugs were administered by rapid
iv injection and courses were repeated every 4 weeks.
Eight patients entered the trial with the following pretreatment characteristics: seven males and 1 female, 7
squamous cell carcinomas and 1 parotid adenocarcinoma,
median age 53 years (43-72), median performance status 75
(50-90). All patients had normal renal and hepatic function. Two had received prior chemotherapy which did not
include MTX or MMC.A total of 20 courses were administered at daily doses ranging between 6 and 10 mg/m2 for MMC
and between 33 and 50 mg/m2 for MTX. Myelosuppression was
the main toxic effect. Five patients entered the trial at
the highest dose level: MMC 10mg/m2 and MTX 50mg/m2 x 2.
The first course was nontoxic in 2, moderately toxic in 1
(1,800 WBC/mm3), and produced life-threatening but reversible myelosuppression in the two remaining patients with
nadir WBC counts of 0 and 100/mm3 respectively and corresponding platelet counts of 600 and 700/mm3. Both were
relatively good-risk patients. On d8, the MTX dose had
been reduced by 50% for leukopenia <3,000/mm3 (2,200 and
2,900 respectively). These 2 patients were subsequently
retreated with 2/3 of the previous toxic doses for 1 and
3 courses respectively: only the second patient presented
myelosuppression, which was rapidly cumulative. Nadir
counts were generally observed at d15 and complete recovery was achieved 1 week later.Other side-effects consisted of minor nausea-vomiting (6/8) and stomatitis (3/8,
severe in 2). No objective antitumor effect could be documented. These findings of excessive and erratic hematologic toxicity make the combination MTX-MMC unattractive
for further investigation.

Institut Jules Bordet, Rue Héger-Bordet,B-1000 Brussels.

22

FEMORAL VENOUS CANNULATION FOR CONTINUOUS ADRIA-
MYCIN (ADR) AND VINDESINE (VDS) INFUSIONS. J.
Bottino, M. Levin, K. Hymes, P. Pouillart, F.
Muggia and B. Nidus. NYU Cancer Center and Fon-
dation Curie, Paris (Study resulting in part from
NCI-INSERM Treatment Research Collaborative
Programs)

ADR and VDS are potent vesicants which to be
given safely by continuous intravenous infusion
require a secure access system. We have investigated femoral vein cannulation as an alternative to superior vena cava catheterization techniques and arteriovenous fistulas or grafts. A
15 cm. Teflon catheter is guided into the femoral
vein over a spring wire which is initially inserted via a 19 gauge needle. A single suture
anchors the unit so patients may ambulate for
short distances. Thirty 24 hr ADR infusions have
been administered to 15 patients without complications. Two of 10 patients given fourteen 48 hr
VDS infusions developed femoral vein thrombosis.
None of the VDS infusions to which hydrocortisone was added was complicated by thrombosis.
We conclude that repetitive femoral vein cannulation is a practical safe method for vesicant
chemotherapy infusions. However, certain drugs
which also regularly cause phlebitis such as
VDS may require special precautionary measures
to reduce the hazard of thrombosis.

NYU Cancer Center, Division of Oncology, 550
First Avenue, New York, NY 10016 U.S.A.

23

CEA IN PANCREATIC JUICE. J. Bourry[1], R. Hayton[2],
C. Bonnet[1], B.Krebs[1], J. Delmont[2]

CEA concentration and flow were assayed in pure pancreatic
juice collected by endoscopic catheterization of the papi-
lla. Pancreatic secretion was stimulated by secretin (1
u/kg) and CCK P2 (3 u/kg); juice was collected in 2-min.
fractions. Volume, CEA concentration (by RIA) and flow
were measured. In several cases CEA values were calculated
before and after centrifugation. 36 patients were studied :
10 pancreatic cancer, 10 chronic pancreatitis (CP), 13
controls (9 with alcohol intake ≥ 75 ml/day (a) and 4 with
<50 ml/day (b)), 3 cancer patients without pancreas in-
volvement.   RESULTS

| | FLOW AFTER: | | CEA CONCENTRATION ng/ml | |
	Secretin	CCK P2	Average	Limits
Panc. cancer	0.95	0.73	419	65.5-860
CP	1.61	1.07	170.9	30-445
Controls:	2.02	2.35		
(a) alcoholic	1.71	2.14	104.67	25-250
(b) non-alcoh.	2.38	2.81	57.25	9-140
Non-pan. cancer	-	-	41	13-80

Juice flow is very low and CEA level high in pancreatic
cancer, but values overlap for the various groups. Centrifugation reduced CEA concentration by 46% in pancreatic
cancer. After CCK, the concentration (+16 to +96%) and
flow (+44 to +75%) rose for CP and controls whereas the
concentration and flow in pancreatic cancer were reduced
by 37% respectively. A dissociation exists between CEA
concentrations in serum and pancreatic juice. Bile presence is accompanied by high CEA values and samples colored
by bile must be excluded. Our results confirm that CEA
in pancreatic juice rises in pancreatic cancer but do not
allow easy separation of such cases from CP. During pancreatic cancer, CEA does not appear to be secreted by the
functional acinus cells of the pancreas as seems to occur
in the other patient groups studied.

Centre A. Lacassagne, 36 Voie Romaine, Nice, France (1) &
Centre d'Hépato-gastroentérologie, CHR, Nice, France (2)

24

PREALBUMIN AND BIOCHEMICAL PROFILE IN CANCER PATIENTS
UNDER PARENTERAL NUTRITION. J.Bourry, G.Milano, C.Caldani,
G.Viot, G.Lesbats, M.Schneider, J.Monticelli, P.Cambon,
C.M.Lalanne

26 cancer patients under parenteral nutrition (PN) (14
men, 12 women) mean age 65.6 years (22-81) were investigated with the following biochemical parameters : Protids
(P), Albumin (Alb), Pre-albumin (Palb), Transferin(Tf),
Retinol Binding Protein (Rbp) and α1 Acid Glycoprotein(Agp).
Mean PN duration was 26.8 days (9-105) , mean energy intake 172.04 kg ^{J}/kg/d (75.33-271.18) and nitrogen intake
0.197 g/kg/d (18-64.8).
Two patient groups were distinguished : Group 1 : clinical
improvement (n=13) - Group 2 : death during or immediately
after PN (n=13). Distribution of mean values at the beginning (B) and during (D) PN was as follows:

| | P g/l | | Alb g/l | | Palb g/l | | Tf g/l | | Rbp 10^3 g/l | | Agp | |
	B	D	B	D	B	D	B	D	B	D	B	D
Group 1	71.3	73.8	26.9	26.6	0.148	0.191	2.05	1.86	47.4	39.1	1.85	1.53
Group 2	69.0	65.9	22.3	22.0	0.110	0.165	1.45	1.54	41.0	51.7	1.99	2.16

All nutritional markers were very low (far from normal
range values) while Agp was elevated, as expected.
Palb appears the most sensitive study marker :
- Levels at the time of starting PN were lower in group 2
than in group 1.
- Correlations between Palb variations and energy and nitrogen intake respectively are positive for group 1
(r = 0.66; r = 0.49).
These coefficients are negative for group 2.
When the nutritional metabolic profile of cancer patients
under PN must be measured, Palb appears to be an interesting parameter with a prognostic value which objectively
reflects energy and nitrogen intake.

Centre Antoine-Lacassagne,36 Voie Romaine, 06054 NICE Cedex

25

RECENT RESULTS WITH NORGAMEM (THIOPROLINE) IN HEAD AND NECK CANCER. A.Brugarolas, M.Gosalvez

Norgamen is the generic name of the chemical compound Thiazolidine-4-carboxylic (also called Thioproline) for its use in cancer clinical trials. This compound was shown by Gosalvez (Biochem.Soc.Trans. 7, 191-192,1979) to induce the restoration of contact inhibition in Hela cells in tissue culture, thus being the first pharmacologic agent able to induce the "reverse transformation" (Puck,T.T., Proc.Natl.Acad.Sci.USA 74,4491-4495,1977) of tumor cells to cells with normal characteristics. Norgamem was brought to a clinical trial in patients with advanced cancer (A.Brugarolas and M.Gosalvez,Lancet,Jan .12,1980,pp 68-70) where it was detected to have anticancer activity, especially in epidermoid carcinoma of the head and neck. Further clinical studies were focused in epidermoid carcinoma of the head and neck defining a subset of sensitive patients among those with well-differentiated histologies. It was observed that those epidermoid head and neck carcinomas not having well-differentiated histologies after progressing under Norgamem therapy, responded, almost in every case, to therapy with Cis-platinum and Bleomycin. The response rate with the combination of Norgamem, Cis-platinum and Bleomycin was significantly much higher than with Cis-platinum and Bleomycin alone in previously treated patients. Additionally, a pilot phase II trial in well-differentiated tumors of long evolution of various histologies and localizations was carried out, and the results indicated that the role of Norgamem in cancer therapy may be wider than anticipated.

Servicio de Oncologia, Hospital General de Asturias, Oviedo and Servicio de Bioquimica Experimental, Clinica Puerta de Hierro, Madrid-35, Spain.

26

PRELIMINARY RESULTS WITH REVERCAN (2-AMINO-2-THIAZOLINE), AN ANALOGUE OF THIOPROLINE, IN BLADDER CARCINOMA. A. Brugarolas[+], A. Usón[++], J.M. Junguera Villa[+] and M. Gosálvez[+++].

Revercan is the name of 2-amino-2-thiazoline chlorhydrate for its use in cancer clinical trials. This compound is an analogue of Norgamem (Thioproline), the first inducer of "reverse transformation" with anticancer activity in the clinics (M. Gosálvez, Proc. AACR and ASCO 20, 17, 1979; M. Gosálvez et al., Biochem.Soc. Trans. 7, 191-92, 1979; A. Brugarolas and M. Gosálvez, Lancet, Jan.12, 1980, pp. 68-70; Puck, T.T., Proc. Natl. Acad. Sci. USA 74, 4491-95, 1977). Revercan was selected by Gosálvez as the only existing derivative of Thioproline which was able to pass the three screening systems for inducers of reverse transformation (M. Gosálvez, Proc. AACR and ASCO 21, 132, 1980) and has been brought to the clinics in Spain in patients with advanced urinary bladder cancer. In 22 evaluable patients with transitional carcinoma of the urinary bladder, Revercan induced 3 biopsy-proven complete tumor remissions and 5 partial remissions for a total response rate of 31%. Tumors with well-differentiated histologies appeared to be more sensitive. Similarly to Thioproline, no toxicity was observed and a broad range of doses and schedules appeared to be equally active. The activity of this derivative of Thioproline further suggests that this new class of compounds may have opened a new way in the therapy of neoplastic disease in man and further investigations are indicated.

Servicio de Oncología and Servicio de Urología, Hospital General de Asturias, Oviedo[+], Departamento de Urología, Hospital Clínico de San Carlos, Madrid[++] and Servicio de Bioquímica Experimental, Clínica Puerta de Hierro, Madrid[+++], Spain.

27

ECHOGRAPHY OF THE THYROID GLAND. J.N.Bruneton, F.Ettore, D.Fenart, M.Abbes, F.Demard, F.Lapalus

Two hundred thyroid lesions were examined by echography following scans and prior to surgery. In 60 cases, a hyperechoic pattern was observed in comparison with normal tissue. In our series, this echographic pattern was always associated with a benign lesion (functionally active vesicular adenoma, benign nodular hyperplasia). The 16 cases of cancer observed all generated a hypoechoic pattern as compared with healthy thyroid tissue. The majority of adenomas also presented a hypoechoic pattern, and in such cases preoperative diagnosis of the benign or malignant nature of the lesion is impossible. Subacute thyroiditis and Riedel's thyroiditis also presented a hypoechoic pattern (9 cases).
Cysts (16 cases) were easily recognized correctly by echography.
In contrast, in cases of goiter, the only value of echography is precise measurement of the size of the thyroid gland since the lesions' heterogenic appearance prevents diagnosis of whether or not neoplastic degeneration has occurred.
The diameter of the smallest nodule detectable with a 5 MHz transducer is 0.5 cm.
As revealed by these findings, echography provides valuable preoperative information in over one third of all cases (hyperechoic nodule, cyst). Echography of the thyroid gland is thus an examination warranting more extensive utilization as part of pre-therapy investigations of thyroid nodules.

Centre Antoine-Lacassagne, 36 Voie Romaine, 06054 Nice Cedex, France

28

SEPARATION OF HUMAN BREAST CANCER CELLS R. Buckman, D. Dearnaley, R.C. Coombes and A.M. Neville

In order to characterise the cell surface of breast cancer cells in different metastatic sites, we have examined several ways of obtaining homogeneous or highly enriched populations of malignant cells. We have examined the following methods (a) plastic plates coated with antibody (b) Percoll gradients, and (c) rosetting of white cells using sheep red cells and 2D1 mouse monoclonal antibody.
Results indicate that separation on discontinuous Percoll gradients followed by rosetting yields highly enriched populations of cancer cells. This technique is now being used to separate malignant breast epithelial cells from biopsies of a variety of sites, and labelling by lactoperoxidase-catalysed radio-iodination is being carried out.

Ludwig Institute for Cancer Research, (London Branch), Unit of Human Cancer Biology, Royal Marsden Hospital, Sutton, Surrey SM2 5PX

8

29

FIVE YEAR FOLLOW-UP OF FAC-BCG ADJUVANT THERAPY OF STAGE II AND III BREAST CANCER. Buzdar, A.U., Blumenschein, G.R., Hortobagyi, G.N., and Yap, H.Y.

Two-hundred and twenty-two patients with stage II and III breast cancer were treated with combination chemoimmuno-therapy following regional therapy. The treatment included Adriamycin 40 mg/m^2 IV Day 1, Cyclophosphamide 400 mg/m^2 IV Day 1 and 5-FU 400 mg/m^2 IV Day 1 and 8 of each 28 day cycle. Upon reaching a 300 mg/m^2 of Adriamycin, Methotrexate was substituted for Adriamycin. Total treatment period was 2 years. BCG was administered by scarification on Days 9, 13 and 17. With median follow-up of 54 months (minimum 38 months, longest 72 months) of patients with stage II disease, 81% of 1-3 node premenopausal patients and 72% of $\geq$4 node premeno-pausal patients remained free of disease. Eighty-five percent of 1-3 node postmenopausal and 69% of $\geq$4 node postmenopausal patients remained free of disease with stage II cancer. Stage III cancer 59.4% of premenopausal patients remained free of disease and 56.8% of postmeno-pausal patients remained free of disease. The toxicity of the treatment has been acceptable. Compliance with treatment was excellent. These results demonstrate that this Adriamycin-containing combination therapy is effective in preventing recurrent disease in both pre and postmenopausal patients with stage II and III breast cancer.

The University of Texas System Cancer Center M. D. Anderson Hospital and Tumor Institute, Houston, Texas 77030 U.S.A.

30

CIRCULATING IMMUNE COMPLEXES IN MONOCLONAL GAMMOPATHIES. * J.P. Cassuto, ** J.F. Quaranta, ** R. Maiolini, * J. Laversanne, ** R. Masseyeff

The incidence of circulating immune complexes (CIC) in monoclonal gammopathies was studied in 61 patients com-prising 27 myelomas and 32 monoclonal gammopathies of un-determined significance (MGUS).
Three methods were used in all these patients : i) poly-ethylene glycol precipitation (PEG test) followed by an immunonephelometric assay of IgG, IgM and C$_4$ of serum and precipitate ; ii) enzyme-immunoassay of CIC (EIA/CIC) by inhibition of a polyclonal rheumatoid factor (RF) ; iii) enzyme-immunoassay of RF (EIA/RF).
Results show that the incidence of CIC is high in both situations : 79.3 % and 65.6 % with PEG test and 55.2 % and 43.7 % with the EIA/CIC respectively for myeloma and MGUS. 17 sera present CIC only by one of the two technics. No RF specific CIC was found in these samples by EIA/RF. Neither the immunoglobulin class nor the presence of renal insufficiency changes the incidence of CIC. Conversely the type of light chain influences this inci-dence : 86.6 % and 71.4 % by PEG test and 60.0 % and 50.0% by EIA/CIC respectively for lambda and kappa chains in myelomas. The observation of anomalous results may be in-terpreted either as the result of the actual occurrence of CIC (however the corresponding antigens remain unknown) or as interferences due to the specific nature of monoclonal immunoglobulin (i.e. enhanced Fc interaction).
In practice, these results show that CIC are more frequent in myeloma than in MGUS but the search for CIC does not represent a discriminative test on the individual basis, or a criterion of renal failure.

* Clinique Médicale (Pr. P. Audoly), CHU, 06031 Nice Cédex
** INSERM FRA 12, Laboratoire d'Immunologie du CHU, 06034 Nice Cédex

31

COMPARATIVE DISTRIBUTION OF ^{57}CO-BLEOMYCIN, ^{67}GA-CITRATE AND ^{167}TM-CITRATE IN MURINE TUMOR AND IN TRANSPLANTED HUMAN TUMOR IN NUDE MICE. J.F.Chatal, E.Diez, D.Guihard, C.Cimetière and J.Léger.

The tumoral tropism of ^{167}Tm-citrate was compared with that of ^{67}Ga-citrate and ^{57}Co-Bleomycin in a murine tumor model (Lewis Lung tumor, C$_{57}$B1$_6$ strain) and in a histolo-gically related human tumor heterotransplanted in a nude mouse. The ^{167}Tm-citrate was produced by ^{167}Er (p,n) ^{167}Tm reaction. For the Lewis Lung tumor, uptake was greatest with ^{167}Tm-citrate at 24 hrs (4.14% dose/g vs 2.86% with ^{67}Ga-citrate and 0.64% with ^{57}Co-Bleomycin). Blood clea-rance of ^{167}Tm-citrate was slower than that of ^{57}Co-Bleomy-cin but appreciably faster than that of ^{67}Ga-citrate. These comparative kinetic studies indicate that the tumor to blood ratio for ^{167}Tm-citrate is much greater than that for ^{67}Ga-citrate and approximately the same as that for ^{57}Co-Bleomycin. The same is true for tumor-to-other-tissue (muscle, intestine, skin) ratios, except that for bone ^{167}Tm-citrate concentration is higher than for the other two radionuclides. For the human tumor, ^{67}Ga-citrate up-take was greater than that of ^{167}Tm-citrate (8.91% dose/g vs 1.51% at 24 hrs), but as the blood clearance of ^{167}Tm-citrate is considerably faster than that of ^{67}Ga-citrate the tumor to blood ratio remained greater for ^{167}Tm-citra-te (28 vs 3 at 24 hrs).
It would thus appear that in the two models studied ^{167}Tm-citrate is superior to ^{67}Ga-citrate and even to ^{57}Co-Bleo-mycin with respect to tumoral uptake and, especially, to the ratios of tumoral activity to that of the other tissues conditioning scintigraphic contrast. As ^{167}Tm-citrate also has favorable radiophysical characteristics (half-life, photon energy), it would be desirable to confirm its poten-tial diagnostic advantages by clinical study, but at pre-sent such study is limited because of the radionuclide's very high production cost.

FRA 13 INSERM- UER de Médecine- 44035 NANTES CEDEX, France

32

NEGATIVE LIPOSOMES LABELED WITH IN 111 OXINE IN TUMOR BEARING MICE. J.F. Chatal, E. Diez, D. Guihard, R. Pasqualini

Negative liposomes composed of lecithin, cholesterol and dicetylphosphate (molar proportion :7:1:2) were labeled in the lipid layer with In 111 oxine. Some batches were soni-cated at 4°C for a variable time and the free radiotracer was removed by column chromatography. In each experiment the average diameter of liposomes was measured by electron microscopy. The tissue distribution of sonicated and non-sonicated liposomes was studied, in C$_{57}$B1$_6$ mice bearing Lewis Lung tumors, 24 and 96 hrs after injection and com-pared with that of Ga 67 citrate with a view to a potential scintigraphic tumor localization. The results, expressed as percentage of the injected activity per gram of tissue, showed a different distribution according to the size of liposomes. With non-sonicated liposomes (average diameter: 169 nm) the respective uptakes of radioactivity by the tumor and liver were 0.99 and 21.7%/g at 24 hrs, whereas with smaller liposomes (average diameter : 49 nm) the up-take by the tumor increased (2.1%/g) and by the liver de-creased (6.9%/g). At 96 hrs the values remained the same in the tumor, liver and muscle but decreased in the blood and intestine. The tumor to blood ratio and tumor to mus-cle ratio were then respectively 8.7 and 3.2. By compari-son the equivalent ratios with Ga 67 Citrate were, at the same time, 4.2 and 12.1 and the uptake by the tumor was 2.2%/g. The replacement of lecithin by cardiolipin did not change the tissue distribution. An attempt to decrease hepatic uptake by injecting large empty liposomes 2 hrs before sonicated labeled ones was unsuccessful.
We conclude that small negative liposomes are potential diagnostic agents as compared with Ga 67 citrate. As an extension of this work we plan the incorporation on to li-posomes of purified antibodies raised against associated tumor antigens in an attempt to increase specificity for tumor cells.

FRA 13 INSERM- UER de Médecine, 44035 NANTES CEDEX- France

33

PROGNOSTIC VALUE OF HORMONE RECEPTOR IN OPERABLE BREAST CANCER. F. Cheix, A. Biron, C. Bailly, E. Pommatau, M. Mayer, S. Saez

The relationship between the estrogen and progesterone receptor (ER, PgR) status and recurrence was examined in 310 women undergoing mastectomy for operable breast cancer.
Their tumors were routinely analysed for estrogen and progesterone cytosol receptors by the dextran-coated charcoal technique using estradiol and R5020 as triated ligands. Relapses were analyzed by the actuarial method.
The distribution of patients who were receptor positive or negative was similar, regardless of several parameters : TNM staging, axillary node status, adjuvant therapy. 47 of 208 ER+ patients recurred with a mean disease free interval (DFI) of 29 months while 23 of 102 ER- patients recurred with a mean DFI of 17.7 months (p < 0.01). In axillary node positive patients, the DFI is 28 months in ER+ patients versus 16.2 months in ER- patients (p < 0.01).
ER and PgR status was known in 151 patients. Among 50 patients with ER+ PgR+ tumors, only one had recurrence (at 23 months), while among 57 cases with ER- PgR- tumors, 10 relapsed after a mean DFI of 17 months.
The difference in recurrence rate is significant (p < 0.01). These data suggest that the use of the two receptors (ER,PgR) may improve the definition of risk of recurrence.

Centre Léon Bérard - 28, rue Laënnec
69373 LYON Cedex 2 - France

34

BINDING OF MEROCYANINE 540 TO HUMAN LEUKEMIC CELLS
C.Choquet, F.Zadra, P.Vaigot, G.Moscati, C.Boucheix, G. Mathé and C. Rosenfeld

Following the technic described by J.Valinsky, T.Easton, E.Reich (Cell 13,487-499,1978)concerning the greater permeability to Merocyanine (MC 540) of leukemic leukocytes compared to the normal cells, we have studied 55 samples of blood of leukemic patients (15 ALL, 17 AML, 9 CML blastic crisis, 3 CLL and 11 LS) and normal donors. Using the flow cytometry technic with a FACS II Cell Sorter, we have measured the fluorescence intensity and the cell size. The data obtained were compared to the following parameters: cytology of peripheral blood and bone-marrow, surface markers, therapy and other clinical data. For some cases, the different populations of cells were separated in function of their fluorescence and their size in order to have morphological controls. In 78% of cases, a good correlation was found between clinical and FACSII data. The small number of discrepancies distributed in the different sub-groups of leukemias does not actually allow to get any eventual significant correlation with the other parameters quoted above. This study is on-going.

ALL:Acute Lymphoid Leukemia, AML:Acute Myeloid Leukemia, CML:Chronic Myeloid Leukemia, CLL:Chronic Lymphoid Leukemia, LS:Lymphosarcoma

This work was supported by grants from CNAMTS, UER Kremlin Bicêtre(782),INSERM (82.79.114)and DGRST(80.7.226)

Département de Culture et de Production de Cellules Humaines, I.C.I.G., I.N.S.E.R.M. U.50, Villejuif, France

35

VINDESINE-CIS-PLATINUM IN ADVANCED MELANOMA. M. Clavel, E. Archimbaud, P. Brun, E. Pommatau

Cis-platinum was shown in a previous study to be an effective agent in advanced melanoma when failure occurs under usual agents. In certain studies, Vindesine has been shown to produce some tumor regression. The combination of CDDP and VDS has been studied in non small cell carcinoma and toxicity was found acceptable.
We initiated a regimen with: Vindesine IV 3 mg/m2 every ten days, and cis-platinum 100 mg/m2 every three weeks. CDDP was administered by 24 hr continuous infusion with mannitol after a day of prehydratation. Nine patients have been treated. All but one of them received previous chemotherapy consisting of DIC and sometimes BLM and CCNU.

N° patients	Failures	Improvement > 50%
9	6	3

Improvement was seen in two cases of pulmonary metastases and in the case reported below:
Mme RAV. - multirecurrent melanoma treated by surgery, DIC, CCNU and Procarbazine with high hematological toxicity. In December 1979 new cutaneous nodes with positive cytological examinations and brain metastases with neurological symptoms were observed. Up until now, complete remission has been obtained without any hematological toxicity. This result on brain metastases raises the problem of drug blood-brain barrier transfer and supports two hypotheses:
- non-bound CDDP may pass through the BBB
- mannitol is able to increase BBB permeability

Centre Léon Bérard, 28 rue Laënnec
69373 Lyon Cédex 2, France

36

CISPLATIN, METHOTREXATE, BLEOMYCIN, VINCRISTINE (CABO) : A PROMISING REGIMEN FOR ADVANCED HEAD AND NECK CANCER. M. Clavel, P. Biron, U. Bruntsch, W. Gallmeier,F. Cavalli, C. Domenge, A. Apchin, F. Conte, J. Michel, J. Vermorken, M. Namer, H. Cortes-Funes, A. Kirkpatrick, J.J. Body and M. Rozencweig.

Fifty-eight pts with squamous cell carcinoma of the head and neck received a combination chemotherapy regimen suitable for ambulatory treatment and consisting of methotrexate 40mg/m2 (d1, 15), cisplatin (C) 50 mg/m2 (d4), bleomycin 10mg (d1, 8, 15) and vincristine (V) 2 mg (d1, 8, 15). Courses were repeated q 3 wks. All drugs were given by iv bolus. C was administered with a 2-hr hydration program. V was withdrawn after the first 2 courses. In this interim analysis, 22 pts were evaluated for response: all were males with a median age of 55 yrs (35-73) and a median performance status (PS) of 80 (60-100).All but one had unresectable cancer: 9 had no prior therapy and 12 had been previously treated with radiotherapy. None of the pts had received any of the 4 drugs included in this regimen.There were 5 complete responses (CR) and 9 partial responses (PR)(>50%), for an overall response rate of 64%. All untreated pts achieved remission (3CR, 6PR).The median response duration was 14+ wks (6+ -39). Toxicity could be evaluated in 32 pts. Leukopenia was the most frequent toxic effect. WBC <4000/mm3 were observed in 26 pts but only 9 had WBC <2000/mm3. Mild thrombocytopenia was noted in 7 pts.Other toxic effects included nausea-vomiting (22),alopecia (16),neurological manifestations (13),infection (8), stomatitis (7), respiratory toxicity (6),fever-chills (5), asthenia (4),cutaneous toxicity (3), and renal impairment (2). Although CABO was tested in a nonrandomized trial, these preliminary results seem very favorable as compared to data obtained with other chemotherapy programs in various cooperative trials. CABO is generally well tolerated in pts with high PS. Full assessment of this regimen must await a final analysis of the trial.

EORTC Head and Neck Cooperative Group.

37

A NEW CASE OF STEWART-TREVES SYNDROME. M. Clavel, J.Y. Bobin, B. Salles, B. Fontaniere, C. Bailly, E. Pommatau

Three cases of Stewart-Treves syndrome have been observed at the Centre Léon Bérard; two have already been published and a new case involving a 52 year old patient is now reported. The patient underwent left mastectomy with axillary node dissection for undifferentiated carcinoma (T2N+) in 1970. Surgery was followed by irradiation. Six months later lymphoedema of the homolateral upper limb appeared, with no modification during eight years. In October 1978, hemorrhagic nodosities had grown on the back of the hand. During the two months necessary for the diagnosis of sarcoma, the lesions had spread over the entire upper limb and onto the thoracic wall drawing the fields of irradiation.
Neither chemotherapy using Adriamycin, DTIC, Vincristine, Actinomycin, Cytoxan-Adriamycin, CDDP, nor surgery or radiotherapy could prevent the disease from recurring and spreading from this moment on. The patient died in December 1979 with pleural effusion and pulmonary metastases.
Cytological and pathological examinations concluded in favor of angiosarcoma.
The clinical evolution, the delay between mastectomy, lymphoedema and sarcoma and the length of survival and failure to respond to therapy are all usual in this disease.
In this case, angiosarcoma was clearly demonstrated. Tumor evolution occurred in the fields of irradiation. The relation with radiotherapy will be discussed.

Centre Léon Bérard, 28 rue Laënnec
69373 Lyon Cédex 2, France

38

ANTIGRIPPAL VACCINATION [1] IN CHEMOTHERAPY-TREATED PATIENTS
M. Clavel, B. Salles, M.C. Bentejac, G. Larbaigt, E. Pommatau

This study was aimed at determining whether such vaccination is able to protect patients receiving chemotherapy. 25 patients (14 males, 11 females) were studied. All received polychemotherapy for advanced malignant disease. Various tumor localizations and histological types were involved. Two protocols were used: certain patients received one injection of 1 cc while others received a second injection one month later.
Sera are treated with RDE and antibody titers are determined using the classic inhibition test against 4 to 8 haemagglutinating units of each of the prototype strains: A Texas 1/77 (H3 N2), AUSSR 90/77 (H1 N1) and B Hong Kong 8/73. Antibody titers of 1.40 and above are considered protective.
Preliminary results show that approximately 75% (A Texas 77) and 60% (AUSSR 77) of patients immunized with one injection are protected. With a 2-injection schedule, 100% protection is obtained for the two A strains. These results are comparable with those obtained for healthy adults.
45% of patients are protected against strain B regardless of the schedule (1 or 2 injections).
In conclusion, a good level of protection is obtained in such a population, and could be better achieved with a 2-injection schedule.

[1] Vaxigrip Mérieux

Centre Léon Bérard, 28 rue Laënnec
69373 Lyon Cédex 2, France

39

DANAZOL TREATMENT FOR ADVANCED BREAST CANCER.
R.C. Coombes, T.J. Powles.

Danazol ("Danol", Sterling Winthrop), is a synthetic steroid that inhibits gonadotrophin secretion and possesses progestogenic and mild androgenic activity. It also inhibits steroidogenesis. To date it has been given in doses of 300-800 mg daily to 12 pre-menopausal and 37 post-menopausal patients. Response to treatment was judged according to U.I.C.C. criteria and complete or partial responses were obtained in 2/12 (16.7%) and 7/37 (20.6%) and stabilisation in 2/12 (16.7%) and 3/37 (8.1%) in pre- and post-menopausal patients respectively. Response duration ranges from 3-12 months at this time.

Danazol suppressed menstruation in 5/8 pre-menopausal patients who were treated for more than two months. Serum gonadotrophin concentrations fell in 8/9 patients in whom they were measured.

Side effects (flushing, lethargy and fluid retention) were mild and occurred in 12/46 (26%) patients. Transient disturbances of liver function were also seen in some patients.

We conclude that danazol is an effective agent in advanced breast cancer: further studies are being carried out to define its role in patient management and its relationship to steroid receptor status.

Ludwig Institute for Cancer Research in conjunction with the Department of Medicine, Royal Marsden Hospital, Sutton, Surrey, SM2 5PX, U.K.

40

EFFECT OF FLURBIPROFEN ON RESPONSE AND SIDE-EFFECTS OF CHEMOTHERAPY IN ADVANCED BREAST CANCER. R.C. Coombes, I.E. Smith, T.J. Powles

Experimental studies indicate that the prostaglandin-synthetase-inhibitor Flurbiprofen ("Froben": Boots) can potentiate the anti-tumour effect and reduce the side-effects of chemotherapy. A randomised trial has, therefore, been carried out in which patients with advanced breast cancer received either Flurbiprofen 100 mg x 3 daily or placebo in addition to conventional Adriamycin/Vinca alkaloid chemotherapy. To date, 50 patients have been assessed.

As assessed by U.I.C.C. criteria, the overall response rate was 81% and 60% in patients receiving Flurbiprofen or placebo respectively. Survival at time of last assessment was 71% for Flurbiprofen-treated as compared to 58% for controls.

Regimen (No. of Patients)	Response Category			
	CR	PR	NC/PD	Overall
VA (23)	7 (30%)	7 (30%)	9 (40%)	60%
VA (27) Plus Flurbiprofen	5 (19%)	17 (62%)	5 (19%)	81%

Significant leukopenia occurred with 63% of flurbiprofen-treated patients compared with 70% of controls.

Since last analysis, a total of 75 patients have been randomised in this study and survival data of the entire group will be presented together with details of bone marrow toxicity in the two treatment groups.

Ludwig Institute for Cancer Research in conjuction with the Department of Medicine, Royal Marsden Hospital, Sutton, Surrey, SM2 5PX, U.K.

41

CLINICAL EVALUATION OF SANDWICH TYPE ENZYME IMMUNOASSAY OF PROSTATE-SPECIFIC ACID PHOSPHATASE. E.H. Cooper, R. Glashan, M.R.G. Robinson & K. Trautner.

A sandwich type ELISA assay for PSAP, developed by Drs.G. Grenner & R.Schmidtberger at the Behringwerke AG, Marburg, Germany has been used in urological practice.

Well controlled prostatic cancer has a level of PSAP <2 ng/ml, approximately 90% are <1 ng/ml; other diseases not involving the prostate had a 95th percentile of <1 ng/ml. Any trauma to the prostate, catheters, acute retention can cause a transient rise of PSAP.

The assay has a high reproducibility and is most useful for detecting changes in the 1-10 ng/ml range. Above this level the enzyme and immunoassays are correlated but the slopes can differ from one laboratory to another.

Longitudinal studies over 2 years indicate controlled patients tend to have very stable PSAP levels. The rate of rise of PSAP tends to be logarithmic with 3-4 months passage through 1-10 ng/ml zone.

The percentage distribution of PSAP levels in untreated patients was :

	n	<2 ng/ml	2.1-10 ng/ml	>10
T1-2 Nx Mo	26	57.7	38.8	3.5
T3-4 Nx Mo	30	46.6	33	20.4
T1-4 Nx M_1	36	8.6	22	69.4

The probability of having a value >3 ng/ml and rising at various times after starting treatment was assessed.

6 months-1 year: Mo $3/_{22}$, M_1 $12/_{23}$; 1-2 years: Mo $0/_{14}$, M_1 $7/_{15}$; and at 3 years: Mo $2/_9$, M_1 $4/_7$.

Unit for Cancer Research, University of Leeds, England.

42

INTEREST OF LONG TERM RIGHT ATRIAL CATHETERIZATION IN ONCO-HEMATOLOGIC PATIENTS. J.Y. Coquin, D. Maraninchi, J.A. Gastaut and Y. Carcassonne

Peripheral venous problems are among the major complications occurring in the treatment of cancer patients. Use of a central vein allows multiple blood examinations, continuous infusion of caustic drugs and parenteral nutrition even in the treatment of outpatients. We evaluated the inocuity and usefulness of the method in 61 patients (32 males, 29 females), mean age 43 $\pm$ 16 years. Seventy catheterizations were performed in these 61 patients; 45 patients had acute leukemia, and there were 16 other malignancies. In 27 patients, parenteral nutrition was performed during chemotherapy. A flexible silicone catheter (VYGON N° 2180-20) was inserted in the jugular vein following surgical disclosure under local anaesthesia. The catheter was then tunneled under the skin until located 10 cm under the clavicule. After an X-ray check, the tip of the catheter was maintained in the right atrium. Blood monitoring, chemotherapy, transfusions and parenteral nutrition were done only in this central line. For outpatients, the connecting portion of the catheter was closed after heparinization - twice a week. Catheterization was maintained during 52 $\pm$ 24 days (4 - 180 days) corresponding to 3000 days of perfusion. Catheter removal was done in 57 patients at the end of treatment, in 5 patients at death, in 6 patients during accidental output, and in 2 patients during infection. 13 outpatients kept this catheter between 30 and 180 days without problem. Incidents during catheterization were minimal: 4% tip infection in patients with sepsis, 10% hepatomas (only in patients with disseminated intravascular coagulation during acute leukemia). The procedure seemed safe and comfortable to the patients and the nursing team. The safety and comfort of this method invite wide use in all intensive cancer treatments.

Institut Paoli-Calmettes, Unité de Nutrition Clinique des Maladies du Sang, Marseille, France

43

THE TREAMENT OF ADVANCED SEMINOMAS WITH CISPLATIN, VIN-BLASTINE AND BLEOMYCIN (PVB). H. Cortés Funes, A. Moyano, A. Manas, C. Mendiola, P. Aramburo

Eleven patients with advanced seminomatous tumors were treated with a combination of Cisplatin, Vinblastine and Bleomycin at doses and on a scheme reported previously (Proc. Eur. Soc. Med. Oncol., 53, p 14, 1979). There were 5 testicular, 2 ovarian and 4 primary mediastinal tumors. Four patients were resistant to previous radiation therapy. The other 7 patients had no prior therapy. All were evaluable for response and toxicity.
The overall response rate was 100% with 9/11 CR and 2/11 PR. Two of the original CRs relapsed at 9 and 12 months. The two PR patients are still under treatment. The other 7 CRs continued without treatment for a follow-up period of 7+ to 23+ months. The response rate was independent of location of the primary. General toxicity was similar to the entire group of germ cell tumors reported on previously. The median follow-up for all patients was 12.5 months.
From this data we can conclude that PVB is an effective regimen for any type of germ cell tumor, including seminomas, giving a high CR rate in advanced disease.
On the basis of this effectiveness, we must consider this chemotherapy not only for relapsed patients but also for the primary therapeutic approach of high risk patients with or without radiation therapy.

Seccion Oncologia Médica, Hospital "1° de Octubre" Madrid, Spain

44

CHEMOTHERAPY OF ADVANCED HEAD AND NECK CANCER WITH HIGH DOSES OF CISPLATINUM AND BLEOMYCIN INFUSION. H. Cortés-Funes, A. Ramos, R. Quiben, C. Mendiola, A. Manas.

Forty-seven patients with advanced head and neck epidermoid carcinomas were treated with combined Cisplatinum and Bleomycin chemotherapy. Cisplatinum was given at a dose of 120 mg/m2 after prehydratation, with mannitol diuresis, in one hour infusion the first day. Posthydratation for fluid replacement followed during 12 hours. Bleomycin at 30 mg, total dose, was given by continuous 24 hour intravenous infusion during five consecutive days immediately after posthydratation.
Twenty-six previously untreated patients with local advanced or bad prognosis tumors (pyriform sinus) received two cycles of this chemotherapy before radical radiation therapy. The other 21 had failed prior irradiation & received the same chemotherapy until response or progression. All 47 patients were evaluable for tumor response and toxicity.
The response rate in previously treated patients was 47.6 % with only one CR in an overall median duration of response of 5.1 months. The patients with no prior therapy had an overall response rate of 65.3 % with 2 CR. In this group of patients after radiation therapy there were 9 CR and 12 PR with an overall response rate of 80.7 % and a median duration of response was not reached.
Toxicity included nausea and vomiting in all patients, alopecia (80 %) fever (76.5 %) skin rash (34 %) WBC less than 2000 (14.4 %) platelets less than 100000 (8.5 %), creatinine clearance below 50 ml/min (6.3 %) with one acute renal failure with death and one acute toxic hepatitis due to Cisplatin.
This result suggests that this regimen may be superior to single agents in head and neck tumors only in patients without previous treatment.

Seccion Oncologia Medica, Hospital "1° de Octubre", Madrid (Spain).

45

CORRELATION BETWEEN ESTROGEN RECEPTORS AND BODY WEIGHT IN
WOMEN WITH BREAST CANCER.
A.N.Critselis, E.J.Carson, L.M.Autuoro, P.Vasallo,D.Brock-
meyer.

Obesity has been linked to an increased risk of breast
cancer and to a poor prognosis. Conversely, the presence
of estrogen receptors (ER) in the tumor appears to be a
positive prognostic indicator. The correlation between body weight (BW) and the presence of ER in breast cancer patients is investigated in this study.

Tumor specimens obtained from 237 women treated by radical
or modified radical mastectomy for breast cancer (stage I
or II) were subjected to ER analysis. All determinations
were performed in duplicate by the dextran-coated charcoal
binding assay (positive 10 fmoles/mg cytosol protein).Pa-
tients were stratified according to BW (above or below 150
lbs) and menstrual status (pre- and post-menopausal), and
their charts were reviewed retrospectively.

Estrogen receptors were identified in 58 of 99 women over
150 lbs (58.6 %) and in 78 of 138 women below 150 lbs
(56.5 %), this difference being not significant. Moreover,
the presence of ER in either of the two BW categories was
not affected by the menstrual status of the patients.

Table.BW and ER in 237 women with breast cancer.

BW Group	Total	Premenopausal	Postmenopausal
>150 lbs	58/99 (58.6%)	10/18 (55.6%)	48/81 (59.3%)
<150 "	78/138(56.5%)	21/34 (61.8%)	57/104(54.8%)

These preliminary data suggest that there is no correlation between ER positivity and obesity. However, any
possible interaction between them in determining the natural history of the tumor and/or the survival of the patients warrants further investigation.
Department of Surgery, Maimonides Medical Center - SUNY,
Downstate Medical Center (4802 10th Ave.,Brooklyn.N.Y.
11219,U.S.A.

46

INTRACELLULAR pH IN HUMAN BREAST CANCER TISSUES:
CORRELATION WITH ESTROGEN AND PROGESTERONE RECEPTORS.
A.N.Critselis, C.P.Carvounis, E.J.Carson, L.M.Autuoro
Information on the intracellular pH (pHi) of human breast
cancer is minimal, although manipulations of the pHi of tu
mors may enhance their susceptibility to radio-and possibly chemotherapy. The purpose of this study was the determination of the pHi of human breast cancer and its correlation with its estrogen (ER) and progesterone (PgR)recep-
tor content, a valuable predictor of the response to hormonal therapy and possibly to other methods of treatment.

Specimens obtained from 19 women treated by modified radical mastectomy for stage I or II breast cancer were subjected to pHi determination and steroid receptor analysis.
The pHi was measured by the distribution of ^{14}C-DMO in the
extra-and intra-cellular water.Steroid receptor determinations were performed by the dextran-coated charcoal binding assay.All determinations were performed in duplicate.

The pHi of the breast cancer tissues studied was 6.60+.04
(Table).It was lower in the specimens with ER/PgR activi-
ty(Group A),than in those without it (Group B).However,
this difference was not significant (p<0.10).

Table:pHi,ER,PgR in breast cancer(mean value+ SEM)

Group	N	pHi	ER	PgR
Total	19	6.60 + 0.04		
Group A	8	6.52 + 0.07	176.4 + 56.6	134.6 + 60.7
Group B	11	6.65 + 0.03	0	0

These preliminary data define the pHi of human breast cancer and suggest a possible association between it and the
presence of steroid receptors.This line of inquiry warrants
further investigation:it may provide valuable information
relating to the prognosis and treatment of breast cancer.

Department of Surgery, Maimonides Medical Center (4802,10th
Ave.,Brooklyn,N.Y.11219)-State University of New York-Down-
state Medical Center,and Department of Medicine,SUNY-Stony
brook,N.Y.,U.S.A.

47

SEX STEROID ACTIVITY ON LEUKEMIC CELLS?   L. Danel,
E. Escrich, D. Diere, D. Hollard, S. Saez

Some evidence of steroid activity on hemopoietic cells is
known to occur. It is well established that glucocorticoids
have a cytolytic effect on lymphoid cells.Androgen derivatives promote prolonged remissions when administered as
adjuvant therapy in acute non-lymphoblastic leukemia (non
ALL).Generally speaking, sex hormones may play a role in
the modulation of the immune response. However, it is not
known whether this therapeutic response to sex steroids
in non-ALL represents effects controlled by a non-recep-
tor mediated mechanism, or represents direct or indirect
effects controlled by specific sex steroid receptors.
Sex steroid binding capacity has been investigated in malignant cells from 32 patients with non-ALL and 30 patients
with ALL. The techniques used for measuring receptors were
similar to those used for measuring estrogen receptors in
breast carcinoma. Specific binding sites of labeled dexamethasone,androgen,estrogen and progestin have been characterized either by competition in cytosol fraction or whole
cell incorporation.In some cases,further characterization
of receptor complex was attempted on sucrose gradient or
sepharose 4B column.Data analysis shows as in the literature that frequency of cases containing dexamethasone receptors is significantly higher in ALL than in non-ALL
and the content of receptors is similar in both sexes. The
distribution of receptors for androgen,estrogen and progestin is similar in the two types of leukemia.No difference was found in relation to sex of the patients. However, in quantitative terms,sex steroid receptors are,when
present,more abundant in males than females.Furthermore,
the content of receptors for steroids in each disease is
significantly different. Indeed, the presence of specific
binding sites for these steroids does not"per se" indicate
a definite relationship between these sites and the therapeutic effect of the sex steroids.

L. DANEL. Centre Léon Bérard 28 rue Laënnec 69008 LYON
France

48

HISTOCHEMICAL IDENTIFICATION OF SEX-STEROID RECEPTORS IN
HUMAN BREAST CANCER. A. Danguy, G. Leclercq, G. Pattyn,
and J.C. Heuson

Search for cytoplasmic and nuclear estradiol (E$_2$) and progesterone (Pg) binding sites was analysed in 50 samples of
human breast cancer with fluorescent labeled steroids.
Fluorescein isothiocyanate (FITC)-labeled bovine serum
albumine (BSA) linked to E$_2$ in position 6 and tetramethyl-
rhodamine (TMRITC)-labeled BSA linked to Pg in position 11
were used.
Frozen sections were incubated for two hours at room temperature with the fluorescent steroids. Intense cytoplasmic and nuclear staining was observed in a significant
proportion of epithelial cells. Furthermore, both E$_2$ and
Pg derivatives displayed a considerable cellular heteroge-
neity in the intensity of fluorescence. Moreover most
positive cells for E$_2$ were also positive for Pg.
The specificity of this labeling was analysed. It was
found that neither compound stained tissue sections
of intestinal tract which was prepared as negative control.
BSA-FITC (without steroid) also failed to stain estrogen
receptor positive breast cancer. These data are consistent with a specific binding. Nevertheless, in several
tumors addition of E$_2$-BSA or Pg-BSA conjugates prior to
the fluorescent conjugates casts some doubt on this conclusion : only a partial decrease in intensity was observed.
Finally the degree of cytoplasmic and nuclear staining was
assessed according to the relative proportion of fluorescent cells. Comparison of this quantitative histochemical
assessment with the chemical ER determination failed to
yield a parallel relationship. The significance of this
discrepancy remains to be elucidated.

Supported by Grants from the "Fonds Cancérologique de la
C.G.E.R." and the "F.R.S.M." (Belgium).

Laboratory of Histology, Faculty of Medecine, 97 rue aux
Laines, B-1000 BRUSSELS, Belgium.

49

RADIOIMMUNOASSAY OF PROSTATIC ACID PHOSPHATASE IN PROSTATIC CANCER.
A.Daver, J.L.Tellier, F.Lavenet, P.Peuvrel, J.F.Chatal.

Radioimmunoassay of prostatic acid phosphatase (PAP) was performed (using the kit from Clinical Assays, Boston USA) on 72 reference subjects, 66 patients with benign hyperplasia, 123 untreated prostatic cancer patients, 55 non-prostatic cancer patients and 42 women.
Mean concentration of PAP in non-acidified serum was 1.3 ± 0.4 ($M\pm SD$) ng/ml for reference subjects and 1.6 ± 0.7 for the group with benign hyperplasia. Consequently, the upper discriminative level for diagnosis of prostatic carcinoma was set at 3 ng/ml. Thus, the overall positive rate for untreated prostatic cancer (all stages combined) was 61% (75/123). The number of cases above 3 ng/ml was 15% for stage A (3/20), 26% for stage B (8/31), 59% for stage C (10/17), and 98% for stage D (54/55). For non-prostatic cancer the positive rate was 4% (2/55). The highest level for women group was 1.6 ng/ml.
Radioimmunoassay was compared with measurement of enzymatic activity in 34 untreated cancer cases (all stages combined). When both assays were performed in the same sampling and optimal storing conditions, the radioimmunoassay was abnormally elevated in 10/12 (83%) as compared to 8/12 (67%) for the enzymatic technique. In contrast, in routine conditions, the positive rate was 77% (17/22) for the radioimmunoassay and 36% (8/22) for the enzymatic test. It would thus appear that radioimmunoassay is more reliable than measurement of enzymatic activity which is lost rapidly.
We can conclude that the test has no value in   early prostatic cancer diagnosis. In contrast, the specificity is very satisfying and the sensibility in metastasis diagnosis is very elevated. The time course study is now in progress for the survey of prostatic cancer treatment and the possible correlation between the PAP level, the stage and the pelvic lymphatic histological involvment.

G.E.R.C.O., rue Moll- 49000 ANGERS, France.

50

NEUROLOGICAL DISORDER IN BREAST CANCER PATIENTS.
D. Dearnaley, D. Kingsley, J. Husband, R.C. Coombes and A.M. Neville

This paper describes a retrospective study of the natural history, clinical features and investigation of 62 breast cancer patients presenting with neurological abnormality suggestive of intra-cerebral metastases over a 2 year period. All patients had computed tomography (CT) of brain and 31 had Technesium brain scans as well. Cerebrospinal fluid (CSF) was examined in 25 patients and histological confirmation of intra-cranial tumour was available to 9. A prospective study was undertaken to determine the value of CSF carcinoembryonic antigen (CEA) estimations in 39 patients with metastatic breast cancer.
Intra-cerebral relapse (17 patients) was an early manifestation of metastatic disease. Multiple tumour deposits were identified in 8 patients by CT, but not by Tc brain scan. Small size (5cm or less on corrected CT) of metastases, whether single or multiple, correlated with good clinical response to treatment. Meningeal carcinomatosis was present in 13 patients, occurring after treatment for widespread disease in 12. Prognosis was poor. Detection was unreliable by CT or Tc brain scan. CSF showed malignant cells in 5 out of 9 cases only on first examination. CEA estimation in CSF was found to improve the diagnostic yield, but levels were also raised in some patients with extensive spinal deposits. Extra-dural deposits underlying skull metastases were responsible for neurological symptoms in 5 patients. Twenty seven patients had no evidence of intra-cranial metastases on follow-up, all had normal CT scan but Tc scan was equivocal in 4 of the 11 studied.
Technesium brain scans will detect most symptomatic intracerebral metastases from breast cancer. CT is necessary to define multiple deposits and is useful as a prognostic index. The detection of early meningeal involvement is unsatisfactory.
Ludwig Institute for Cancer Research,(London Branch),Unit of Human Cancer Biology, Royal Marsden Hospital, Sutton, Surrey SM2 5PX

51

USE OF MYCOBACTERIUM SMEGMATIS AS AN IMMUNOSTIMULANT AFTER RESECTION OF LUNG CARCINOMA. G.Decroix, D.Fichet, B.Asselain, C.Chastang.
A randomised trial (Compendium of Tumor Immunotherapy Protocols, registry n°0525) compares the natural history of resected lung carcinoma with a programme of post-operative non-specific immunotherapy using   heat-killed saprophytic mycobacteria: M.smegmatis ATCC 607. From March 1, 1978 to Jan. 1, 1980, 165 patients were entered into the trial. They were randomised in five medical centers, 81 in the control group receiving no treatment, 84 in the immunotherapy group. Information on patients' immunological status was obtained through skin testing with recall antigens (tuberculin, streptococcus, tricophyton, diphtheric and tetanic toxin) and with DNCB.Average age was 59. 91% were males; 91% were heavy smokers, 14% were non-responders to tuberculin skin test. Surgery and pathological staging was as follows : stage IA 15% - stage IB 39% - stage II 21% - stage III 25% (T3 with any N or N2 with any T-M0). The histological findings showed : 72% squamous cell carcinoma - 17% adenocarcinoma - 11% undifferentiated (oat cell excluded). The overall one year survival rate was 75%, 68% in the control group, 82% in the immunotherapy group. The difference is not significant. One year disease free survival is 60% : 57% in the control group and 63% in the immunotherapy group (not significant).
Comparative analysis of TNM classification and staging in relation to survival showed that immunotherapy produced a numerically greater survival rate in each group. None of these figures was statistically significant, except for the patients with mediastinal node involvement where the difference in survival between control and immunotherapy group is borderline (p=0.07). Median survival after recurrence is 2.5 months in the control group and 4 months in the immunotherapy group. Since none of these figures is statistically significant, our study is still open   for patient   entry and must be completed for better evaluation.

Hôpital St Antoine,Service Pneumologie,75571 PARIS Cedex12

52

INCREASED MARROW CFU-$_c$ GROWTH AFTER   4 DAYS STORAGE AT 4°C IN PATIENTS WITH MALIGNANT LYMPHOMA. A.Delforge, E. Rongé-Collard, M.Malarme, M.Mattelaer, T.Spiro and P. Stryckmans

Marrow cells from patients with malignant lymphoma have been shown to contain less CFU-$_c$ (clusters + colonies) than normal marrows (1).
The CFU-$_c$ growth of 29 patients with malignant lymphoma and of 27 normal subjects were compared before (D_1) and after a 4 day stay at 4°C (D_4). In patients with malignant lymphoma the median ratio between the CFU-$_c$ growth at D_4 and D_1 (D_4/D_1) was 1.54, for normals this ratio was 0.9. This increased CFU-$_c$ growth was due to the appearance of more GM CFU-$_c$. Indomethacine 10^{-6}M was added to the lymphoma marrow cells to prevent the synthesis of PGE_2, an inhibitor of   CFU-$_c$ growth; the median ratio of growth in presence of indomethacine over the one obtained without was 1.25.
The inhibitory effect of normal or lymphoma blood lymphocytes (x 0.125 to $2x10^6$/dish) on normal CFU-$_c$ growth were compared; the lymphoma blood lymphocytes did not inhibit the normal CFU-$_c$ growth in a greater fashion than did normal lymphocytes.
These results suggest that an inhibition rather than a loss is responsible for the decreased CFU-$_c$ in the marrow of patients with lymphoma. The inhibition of the CFU-$_c$ growth seen at D_1 in the marrow of lymphoma patients is not due to an increased level of PGE_2 produced by the macrophage or to a stronger inhibiting activity of lymphoma lymphocytes in comparison to normal.
CFU-$_c$: colony forming unit in culture.

1) Bull.J.M., De Vita V.T., Carbone P. Blood 45 : 833, 1975

Service de Médecine et Laboratoire d'Investigation Clinique H. Tagnon, Inst. J. Bordet, Brussels, Belgium

14

53

HEMODIALYSIS AND INDUCTION TREATMENT OF AGGRESSIVE
LYMPHOMAS-LEUKEMIAS. P. Deteix, H. Vu Van, T. Ponchon,
B. Coiffier, P. Tremisi, D. Fiere.

8 patients with tumoral and proliferative lymphomas and
leukemias, and biological features of cellular lysis
syndrome, were treated by urate-oxydase, induction
chemotherapy and hemodialysis. 3 patients (B-ALL, T-ALL,
AML) had initial acute renal failure, at least 2 hemo-
dialyses were performed after chemotherapy, 2 patients
were alive, 1 death was observed in aplasia. 5 patients
(B-ALL, T-Lymphoma, 3 Lymphomas) had no initial acute
renal failure, one hemodialysis was systematically
performed after chemotherapy, no death by cellular lysis
syndrome was observed. 3 patients are alive, 2 died in
aplasia. In aggressive forms of lymphomas-leukemias
chemotherapy can be initiated with renal and metabolic
surveillance, and hemodialysis, in respect of drug
pharmacokinetics, allows efficient treatment.

Services d'Hématologie (Pr Viala) et de Néphrologie
(Pr Traeger), Hôpital E. Herriot, 69374 Lyon - France.

54

IN VIVO AND IN VITRO ASSESSMENT OF HORMONE DEPENDENCE IN
THE MXT MURINE MAMMARY TUMOR. N.Devleeschouwer, D.Gangji,
G.Leclercq and J.C.Heuson

The hormone dependency of the MXT mammary tumor (kindly
provided by D.Medina, Cancer Res. 37, 3344, 1977) was studied in female BD_2F_1 mice. This transplantable tumor contains estrogen receptors (50 fmol/mg protein). Tumor growth
was estimated by measuring the change in tumor surface (TS).
It was slower in ovariectomized than in intact mice (TS at
8 wks, 161 vs 264). This effect was abolished by the s.c.
administration of estradiol (E_2) + medroxyprogesterone acetate (MAP) at the doses of 0.5 μg biw and 0.5 mg qw respectively. The antiestrogen Tamoxifen (TAM) was inhibitory at
doses ranging from 0.5 to 100 mg/kg s.c. biw, with a maximum at 5 mg/kg (TS at 8 wks, 59 vs 264). The antiprolactin
α-bromocryptin (CB 154) (s.c. 25 or 50 mg/kg biw) also
decreased growth (TS at 10 wks, 127 vs 243). Similar results were obtained when these treatments, except CB 154
which was not tested, were applied to 4-wk old established
nodules. In vitro studies were conducted on a cell line
established from MXT in this laboratory and kept for 40
passages as a monolayer in MEM + 15 % fetal calf serum.
TAM ($6x10^{-5}M$) or Nafoxidine ($10^{-5}M$) inhibited cell growth
in vitro. Clonogenic assay in double-layer soft agar was
successful with a cloning efficiency of 15 %. S.c. inocu-
lation of $5x10^5$ cells to the mouse yielded growing tumors
in 80 % of the recipients after a latency period of 4 weeks.
We conclude that MXT provides a useful model for in vivo
and in vitro investigations of hormone dependency of mammary tumors.

Supported by Caisse Générale d'Epargne et de Retraite
(Belgium) and by NCI (U.S.A.) contract n°I-CM-53840.

Service de Médecine, Clinique et Lab. de Cancérologie
Mammaire, Inst. J. Bordet, Brussels, Belgium

55

SERUM COPPER AND IRON LEVELS IN GI-TUMORS. P. Dias Wickramanayake, H.O.Klein

Several authors have found serum copper to be elevated in
pts. with osteosarcoma, Hodgkin's disease, in pregnant
women, and in those on oral contraceptives. Serum Fe levels are generally decreased in pts. with acute infections, pcp, and neoplasms. Our study was undertaken in
3o pts. with histologically proven GI-tumors in different
phases of their disease in order to establish the value
of measurement of serum Cu and Fe in correlation with the
CEA titer and the extent of disease. 12 pts. had gastric,
15 colon and 3 rectum cancer. The pts. age varied between 26 and 78 years. In all pts. the extent of disease
was assessed by physical examination, general blood examination, CEA titer, liver and bone scan, chest film and
axial computer tomography. All pts. had the same cytostatic chemotherapy. The results were compared with those
obtained in 2o age- and sex-matched controls (Cu98-121γ%
- mean 1o7γ %, Fe (16o-2o1γ %, mean 171γ %). The range of
serum Cu and Fe concentration for pts. with GI-tumors in
remission was for Cu 92-14oγ % (mean 112γ %) and for Fe
65-15oγ % (mean 1o5γ %). The range for pts. who did not
respond or those in relapse was for Cu between 17o-3o3γ %
(mean 212γ %) and for Fe between 26-54γ % (mean 31γ %).
All pts. with different histological tumors showed the
same pattern of Cu and Fe concentration according to extent of disease. Statistical analysis (Wilcoxon test)
showed significant difference ($p < 0,005$) for Cu and Fe
concentrations in pts. with relapse and complete remission. Although the number of pts. in this study is relatively small we conclude that the serum Cu and Fe level
is another non-specific and fairly reliable indicator in
GI-tumors to monitor the status of disease, including
detection of early relapse. In a larger study the validi-
ty of these results are proven.

Medical Clinic, University of Cologne, Joseph-Stelzmann-
Strasse 9, 5-5ooo Köln 41 (F.R.G.)

56

PHASE I- AND II-STUDY IN PATIENTS (PTS.) WITH
ADVANCED BREAST CANCER USING A SEQUENTIAL COM-
BINATION OF HIGH DOSE METHOTREXATE (MTX) AND
5-FU. P. Dias Wickramanayake, H.O.Klein, Th.
Löffler

The sequential combination of MTX and 5-FU im-
proves the killing effect in L121o and human
breast cancer cells in vitro if MTX is administered 3-4 hrs. before 5-FU. The reverse of simultaneous injection of both drugs is less active or antagonistic (Cadman et al.,1979; Done-
hover et al.,198o). It was our aim to find out
whether such a combination could cause responses in pts. with progressive breast cancer refractory to conventional chemotherapy. 15 pts.
(Karnofsky 5o-8o%, age 27-68 years) were treated with a bolus injection of MTX (15oo mg/m^2)
and 1 h later with a bolus injection of 5-FU
(15oo mg/m^2). Leucovorin (15 mg q 6 hrs x 3
days) rescue started 24 hrs. after MTX. Hydration (5 l/d i.v.) began 1 day before chemotherapy and continued for further 3 days. Treatment
was repeated every 28 days. Quantitative serum
determinations of MTX were performed by an enzyme immunoassay and HPLC. Between 3o and 48
hrs. after MTX serum concentrations were less
than $1 x 1o^{-7}$ molar in all pts. 6/15 pts.(4o%)
came in PR, 4/15 (27%) had stable disease,4/15
(27%) showed no response. 1/15 (6%) could not
be evaluated. Medium duration of response was 3
months. Nausea and vomiting were tolerable. Renal failure did not occur. In all pts. a transient increase of transaminases and alopecia
were observed. Leukopenia and severe stomatitis
occurred in 9 pts.

Medical Clinic, University of Cologne, Joseph-
Stelzmann-Strasse 9, D-5ooo Köln 41 (F.R.G.)

57

HETEROTRANSPLANTATION OF HUMAN MALIGNANT MELANOMA CELL
LINES IN NUDE MICE. J.F. Doré, R. Jacubovich,
H. Cabrillat[+], and S. Bertrand[++].

10 cell lines established from metastatic human malignant melanoma were heterotransplanted (2.10^6 cells,s.c.)
in outbred nude mice (Iffa-Credo). 7 of these lines gave
50-100% tumor takes within 2 months, but for the 3 other
lines the tumor take never exceeded 25%. However, these
latter lines can grow in irradiated (450r) nude mice
within one week. The i.p. injection of silica particles,
which eliminate phagocytic cells in vivo, results in an
effect comparable to that of a 450r irradiation. The
admixture of BCG (100-500ug, Immuno-BCG Pasteur) to
cells from a line usually giving 80-100% tumor takes in
untreated nude mice reduces the tumor take down to 10-
10%, the effect of BCG being more pronounced when low
numbers of melanoma cells are grafted (10^6). The injection of BCG at a distance from the grafted cells does
not influence tumor take.

Thus, it appears that the nude mouse has the capacity
to reject grafts from some human malignant melanoma
lines, and that the mechanisms involved are susceptible
to irradiation and/or silica and enhanced by BCG
admixed to the grafted cells. Preliminary experiments
tend to indicate that several mechanisms may operate
in the recognition and rejection of human melanoma
heterografts in nude mice.

INSERM FRA 24, [+]Unité de Morphologie Cellulaire et
Tissulaire, and [++]Laboratoire de Cytogénétique,
Centre Léon Bérard, 28 rue Laënnec, 69373 Lyon Cedex 2,
France.

58

POTENTIATION OF AMSA EFFECTIVENESS AGAINST MURINE TUMORS
BY OTHER CARCINOSTATIC AGENTS. P. Dumont and G. Atassi

m-AMSA or methanesulfon-m-anisidide 4'-[9 acridinyl amino]
is an interesting intercalating agent which showed
therapeutic activity in patients with myelogenous acute
leukemia, lymphoma and adenocarcinoma. In the present
investigation on mice, we have compared the therapeutic
activity against L1210 leukemia of the AMSA-melphalan (MLP)-
BCNU (2 + 2.5 + 15 mg/kg), MLP-BCNU-DTIC (2.5 + 15 + 80 mg/kg),
AMSA-DTIC-BCNU (2 + 60 + 15 mg/kg) and AMSA-DTIC-MLP (2 + 80
+ 2.5 mg/kg) combinations. The dose levels of the drugs
used in the combinations were only 30 to 50 % of the
optimal doses of the drugs given separately. The optimal
schedule of treatment was followed for each drug :
days 1-9 for AMSA, days 1,5 and 9 for DTIC and MLP and
day 1 only for BCNU.
The first two combinations proved to be equal and the most
effective of those tested, inducing an increase in lifespan (I.L.S.) of over 200 % with 30 % cures while the
I.L.S. obtained with each drug given alone never reached
more than 100 % or gave cures. The AMSA-DTIC-BCNU combination was less active and yet has shown a good
synergism (I.L.S of 171% and 20 % cures) while the fourth
combination did not show any synergism at any dose
regimen in comparison to the drug given separately. When
DTIC (80 mg/kg X 3) was added to the AMSA-MLP-BCNU combination, a considerable lengthening of survival was
observed (I.L.S.>600 %) and 70 % cures were recorded on
day 90. These results may favour scheduling of clinical
trials with such combinations.

Institut Jules Bordet, Service de Médecine et d'Investigation clinique, Rue Héger-Bordet 1, 1000 Bruxelles, Belgique.

59

CONSOLIDATION AND MAINTENANCE THERAPIES IN ACUTE LYMPHO-
BLASTIC LEUKEMIA. EORTC[*] Hemopathies Working Party

A study was started in 1971 to evaluate the efficacy of
immunotherapy given during complete remission (CR) of
acute lymphoblastic leukemia (ALL). 217 ALL patients in
their first CR were randomized (children and adults separately) to receive for 1 year as consolidation either polychemotherapy (A): successively (L-asparaginase and 6MP),
(6MP and prednisolone), (BCNU and cyclophosphamide) and
(methotrexate and vincristine) or monochemotherapy (B):
methotrexate (MTX) interspersed by reinductions (prednisolone + vincristine). The patients still in CR after one
year were again randomized for maintenance (C) chemotherapy: (6MP +MTX) interspersed by reinductions or maintenance
(I) immunotherapy: fresh BCG (Pasteur Brussels) scarifications and non-irradiated allogeneic ALL blasts.
A regression analysis (Cox's model) indicated that the
level of hemoglobin at diagnosis is a significant prognostic factor. When considering separately the patients treated by consolidation A or B, only those treated by B
showed a significantly better prognosis with a low Hb
(<8 gr Hb/dl).
When considering of the children (< 15 yr) only those with
less than 8 gr Hb, consolidation B (35 patients) gave 77%
survival at 8 years while only 52% survived with consolidation A (45 patients) (p=0.03). With maintenance C (26
patients), 93% were in CR at 8 years versus 53% with I
(25 patients) (p=0.01).
For the patients with >8 gr Hb/dl at diagnosis, since immunotherapy and chemotherapy gave identical results, it is
not possible to ascertain whether they were equally effective or equally ineffective.
We conclude that (1) a patient characteristic can be prognostic or not depending on the treatment administered (2)
the type of ALL producing low hemoglobin at diagnosis
appears highly sensitive to methotrexate and insensitive
to immunotherapy.
* European Organization for Research and Treatment of Cancer (paper presented by P. Stryckmans, Secretary)

60

A,B,H ANTIGENS AND CEA IN BLADDER TUMORS. C. Fella,
J.C. Hammou, J. Vacant

A,B,H antigens, xenoantigens found on a wide scale in our
environment (bacteria, plants, animals), are pluritissu-
lar and are not the result of primary gene transcription.
We employed an original immunofluorescence technique to
reveal the presence of these antigens in histological
sections of both normal and tumoral bladder mucosa.
Highly significant disparities, ranging from conservation
of the antigenic character in all cells to complete loss,
were observed from one tumor to another.
This phenomen is probably due to non-adherence of the
A,B,H blood group substances by the corresponding glyco-
syl transferases to the glycopeptidic backbone.
Carcinoembryonic antigen was demonstrated by immunofluorescence in tumors which had lost all A,B,H blood group
substances.
Study of bladder tumors and bladder mucosa specimens at
a distance has allowed us to draw up a new preliminary
classification system for bladder tumors.

Centre Antoine Lacassagne, 36 Voie Romaine
06054 Nice Cédex, France

61

EVALUATION OF TUMOR MARKERS FOR OPERABLE BREAST CANCER.
J.J.Fennelly, B.Cantwell, T.Ryan, C.Ryan, M.Jones

From 1975 to 1980, 150 patients with operable breast
cancer were studied to evaluate the role of the following
tumor markers :
Serum Alkaline Phosphatase, 5 Nucleotidase, C.E.A., Urinary hydroxyproline, E.S.R., Sialic Acid and more recently
Fucose. Patients were staged according to the U.I.C.C.
method; chest x-ray was carried out every six months and
bone scan once yearly.
Almost all patients with stage II disease received adjuvant chemotherapy; all patients with stage III disease
received adjuvant chemotherapy or hormone therapy plus
radiotherapy.
Experience to date indicates that 50% of patients develop
recurrence without any abnormality of the markers outlined
above, but that at some stage patients who have developed
metastatic disease 75% show an abnormality of one of these
markers.
C.E.A. and Sialic Acid appear to be the most sensitive
markers for the progression of disease; E.S.R. appears
to be non-specific in that it was not necessarily associated with development of metastatic disease though elevated for many months; Serum Alkaline Phosphatase was of
value in 20% of cases; Hydroxyproline was so variable from
day to day that is was difficult to rely on this as a
method of assay.
The most recent data suggests that Fucose is a valuable
parameter of similar sensitivity to that of Sialic Acid.

St.Vincents Hospital, Elm Park , Dublin 4, Ireland

62

A NOVEL ENZYME IMMUNOASSAY FOR METHOTREXATE. B. Ferrua [*]
and R. Masseyeff [*]

An original method using peroxidase labelled rabbit anti-
methotrexate antibodies has been developed to quantify
methotrexate in biological samples. This method is based
on the competition between the methotrexate to be assayed
and the immunogen (methotrexate-bovine serum albumin) phy-
sically adsorbed onto a polystyrene ball, towards a fixed
amount of peroxidase labelled anti-methotrexate IgG.
After washings, the enzymatic activity bound to the ball
was measured using orthophenylene diamine as chromogen.
Methotrexate concentration was a reverse function of ab-
sorbance.
The assay is completed within two hours. The sensitivity
threshold is 0.05 µg/liter or 1.1×10^{-10} M. In the assay
range, which extended from 0.1 to 100 µg/liter, the intra-
assay coefficients of variation varied from 1.5 % to 11.5%.
Up to now, no artifact was noted when calibration curves
were made using different individual sera as diluents. A
main advantage of this technique (which is also applicable
to larger antigen molecules) is that it requires only the
IgG fraction of a specific antiserum, which is easy to
prepare and to label with enzymes using standard procedures, whatever the specificity of the antiserum may be.
Furthermore, the reagents are completely stable, thus
allowing   more convenient utilization than that of
isotopically labelled reagents.

[*] Laboratoire d'Immunologie, FRA 12 INSERM
06034 Nice Cédex

63

COMPARISON OF TWO SCHEDULES OF DRUG ADMINISTRATION IN
ACUTE MYELOID LEUKEMIA. D.Fière, H.Vu Van, B.Coiffier,
O.Gentilhomme, P.A.Bryon, J.J.Viala

Patients with newly diagnosed acute myeloid leukemia(AML)
have been treated for induction remission with oral Thio-
guanine (200 mg/m^2) : hour 0-12, each day for 7 days, and
cytosine arabinoside (200 mg/m^2) with 50 mg by I.V. bolus
followed by 150 mg in continuous infusion : hour 12-24,
each day for 7 days. By randomisation, Daunorubicine
(70 mg/m^2) is added either days 1-2-3 : group A, or days
5-6-7 : group B, by I.V. bolus.
Patients in remission receive intermittent monthly chemotherapy courses with 3 consolidations, 8 maintenances and
3 late intensifications for a period of 15 months.
Another randomisation with B.C.G. or leukemic cells +
neuraminidase vaccination occurs between courses of chemotherapy, during remission.
Between October 1979 and June 1980, 31 patients with AML
entered this protocol : 16 in group A with 14 complete
remissions (C.R.), 2 failures and 2 relapses; 15 in
group B with 11 C.R.s, 4 failures and no relapses.
The overall remission rate is 80% and for group A and
group B respectively 87% and 73%.
Other data and correlations will be discussed.

Service d'Hématologie. Hôpital Edouard Herriot,
69374 Lyon Cedex 2, France

64

KINETICS OF AN ISLET CELL TUMOUR OF GOLDEN HAMS-
TER WITH SPECIAL REFERENCE TO CIRCADIAN VARIABI-
LITY. C. Focan

In an islet tumour of golden hamster exhibiting
a gompertzian type of growth, we performed a kinetic analysis during the 42nd diurnal period
following grafting. The following data were evidenced : (1) variation of mitotic and ^{3}H-TdR labelling indices during the diurnal period (peaks
at noon);(2) variability of mean grain counts of
labelled cells after ^{3}H-TdR (valley at 04.00 and
08.00 hrs);(3) variability of PLM data according
to the hour of ^{3}H-TdR injection (12.00/24.00hrs).
The most striking event was a shift between G_1
and S phase as shown in Table 1.

Table 1. Length of cell cycle phases in islet
cell tumour labelled at different times of day.

Cycle phase	^{3}H-TdR:12.00hours	^{3}H-TdR:24.00 hours
TG_2+M/2(h)	0.95	0.85
TS (h)	14.05	19.40
TG_1+M/2(h)	16.95	11.60
Tc (h)	31.95	31.15

By summing and integrating the data obtained, we
calculated the growth fraction (0.33), the poten
tial doubling time (77.2-92hr) and the cell loss
(0.7).
The importance of circadian fluctuations of proliferation will be discussed not only at the the-
oretical level (interpretation of kinetics in
non-asynchronous systems) but also at the practical level (choice of the time and the sequence
of oncolytic drugs in chemotherapy of experimental and human solid tumours).

University of Liege, Belgium

65

INTEREST OF THE SURVEY OF SERUM MAGNESIUM LEVEL IN
PATIENTS RECEIVING CISPLATIN .

P. Fumoleau, S. Bourdin, P. Peuvrel, B. Le Mével .

Cisplatin (cis-diamminedichloroplatinum II, CDDP) is an
organic compound active against tumors but with high
nephrotoxicity . Renal function impairment has been associated with tubular damage and seems to be cumulative .
Creatinineclearance is usually studied to detect this
renal toxicity ; however, it is known that tubular lesions are not early associated with elevated creatininemia but, rather, with a loss of electrolytes, like
magnesium .
We studied concomitantly creatininemia and magnesemia
in 20 patients before and after each course of CDDP
(100 mg/m2 every 3 weeks, with hydratation and manitol).
Hypomagnesemia (serum magnesium level $<$0.6 mmol/l) was
observed in 5 patients respectively after 3,3,3,4 and 6
courses of chemotherapy . At the same time, creatininemia was normal in all patients ($<$ 12 mg/l).
In 3 of these 5 patients, continuation of the treatment
by CDDP was associated with an increase of creatininemia
($>$ 20 mg/l) after only one additive course, leading to
forced diuresis .
In the 2 other patients, CDDP was stopped and the magnesium level returned to normal value in one month .
We conclude that hypomagnesemia is frequent (5/20) in
patients receiving CDDP . This hypomagnesemia appears
before the increase of creatininemia and seems to be
easily reversible when the treatment is stopped . So it
appears that the dosage of this electrolyte can be used
to detect early signs of tubular nephrotoxicity, and has
to be included in the monitoring of patients receiving
CDDP .

Centre René-Gauducheau (Dir : Pr R. GUIHARD)
Quai Moncousu 44035 Nantes Cedex (France)

66

COMPLETE REMISSION INDUCED BY HIGH DOSE METHOTREXATE
(HDMTX) IN RECURRENT MEDULLOBLASTOMA : REPORT OF 2 CASES

P. Fumoleau, G. Ricolleau, A. Le Mével-Le Pourhiet,
B. Le Mével .

The prognosis of recurrent medulloblastoma is very poor .
Two patients (7 and 10 years old) with recurrent medulloblastoma, after primary treatment by surgery and radiotherapy, were given high dose Methotrexate . Recurrences
were detected by clinical examination and brain scan :
local cerebellar recurrences and carcinomatous meningitis.
The treatment schedule was : vincristine (1,5 mg/m2) followed 6 hours later by MTX (3 g/m2 in 6 hours infusion) ;
citrovorum factor rescue was started 3 hours after . MTX
serum level was monitored by radio-immuno assay (C.I.S.,
Marcoule, France) . Interval between courses was 2 weeks
during the first two months and then 3 weeks ; the dose
of MTX was increased to 4 g/m2 after 2 months .
After 4 courses of high dose MTX, clinical examination
and brain scan showed an apparent complete remission
(C.R.) in the 2 patients . These two C.R. last now for
9 + and 7 + months .
Due to hydratation, alkalinisation and the use of citrovorum factor, we observed no hematologic or renal toxicity . Nausea and mucositis were mild .
MTX levels at 24 hours were always under 10^{-6} mole/l .
We conclude that high dose MTX can be given safely to
children   with recurrent medulloblastoma, with
objective clear remission of their disease .

Centre René-Gauducheau (Dir : Pr R. GUIHARD)
Quai Moncousu 44035 Nantes Cedex (France)

67

DOUBLING TIME AND HORMONE RECEPTORS OF PRIMARY BREAST
CANCER. E.Galante, S.DiPietro, A.Bono, N.Nicoli

The scope of this study was to determine if there is a significant relationship between the doubling time of primary breast cancer and the presence of hormone receptors as
regards both prognosis and therapy. Of 194 cases, for whom
the volumetric doubling time was evaluated from a duplicate mammography performed before surgery, 96 underwent estrogen receptor (ER) determinations. Sixty-five (65.6%)
were ER+, 21 (21.8%) were ER-, and 10 (12.6%) were borderline. The 65 ER+ cases were subdivided as follows : 8
(12.3%) fast, 25 (38.5%) intermediate, and 32 (49.2%) slow.
The 10 borderline cases were subdivided into 2 (20%) fast,
7 (70%) intermediate and 1 (10%) slow. When considered in
relation to the growth rate, the cases were distributed as
follows : fast, 53% ER+, 13% borderline, 33% ER-; intermediate, 59% ER+, 16% borderline, 23% ER-; slow, 82% ER-,
2.5% borderline, 15% ER-. Of the 59 cases with a follow-up
greater than 24 months, 16 had recurrences (regardless of
treatment or N status) : 11 of 44 ER+ (25%) and 5 of 15
ER- (33%). When considered in relation to the growth rate
the cases were distributed as follows : ER+, 2 of 7 (20.8%)
fast, 7 of 19 (36.8%) intermediate, 2 of 18 (11%) slow;
ER-, 2 of 5 (40%) fast, 3 of 8 (37%) intermediate, 0 of
2 (0%) slow.
We conclude that the better course of the ER+ tumors(which
has been widely reported in the literature) is probably
due to the fact that they are comprised of a higher number
of slow growing tumors than are ER- tumors.

Istituto Nazionale per lo Studio e la Cura dei Tumori,
Via Venezian 1, 20133 Milan, Italy.

68

HUMAN CHORIONIC GONADOTROPIN, TESTOSTERONE, LUTEINIZING
HORMONE AND PROLACTIN IN PATIENTS WITH PULMONARY CANCER.
E. Galante, G. Secreto, C. Recchione, V. Dati, A. Zadro,
and G. Ravasi.

The scope was to study, in untreated pulmonary cancer
patients, the existence of higher than normal levels of
human chorionic gonadotropin (HCG), testosterone (TST),
luteinizing hormone (LH) and prolactin (PRL). The hema-
tic levels of these hormones determined by the radioimmunoassay in 59 patients with pulmonary cancer (33 squamous cell carcinomas,16 adenocarcinomas, 5 oat cell carcinomas and 5 undifferentiated, large cell carcinomas),
aged 40 to 73 years, were compared with those of normal
controls within the same age group. Beta-HCG was present
in 4 of 59 cases (6.8 %). The mean LH of 55 cases (exclu-
ding the 4 β-HCG positive cases) was 12.57 + 7.83 compa
red to 8.89 + 3.99 of 32 controls (p< 0.002). The mean
PRL was 12.22 + 6.42 compared to 6.88 + 2.72 of 30
controls (p< 0.001). The mean TST was 4.20 + 1.60 compared to 4.78 + 1.67 of 38 controls (no statistical significance). However, an evaluation of TST values as a function of histologic type showed that N+ squamous cell
carcinomas had a mean value of 2.93 + 1.51 compared to
4.77 + 1.35 for N- squamous cell carcinomas (13 cases),
and this data was statistically significant. In contrast,
there was no difference between the mean value of the
adenocarcinomas and that of undifferentiated large cell
carcinomas. It is concluded that there are significant
variations in the production of LH, PRL and TST in pulmonary cancer patients, particularly in those with squamous cell carcinoma. The values of the production of
β -HCG were the same as those reported in the literature.

Istituto Nazionale per lo Studio e la Cura dei Tumori,
Via Venezian 1, 20133 Milan, Italy.

18

69

ISOLATION OF A HUMAN T CELL LINE Be13 EXPRES-
SING BOTH PROTHYMOCYTE AND THYMOCYTE CHARACTE-
RISTICS AND ATTEMPTS TO INDUCE DIFFERENTIATION
WITH THE PHORBOL ESTER TPA

N. Galili[1], U. Galili[2], Z. Ravid[1], M. Schlesinger[1] and N. Goldblum[1]

A human T cell line was isolated from the bone
marrow of a 7 year old girl in a second relapse
diagnosed as having T-ALL. Like human prothymo-
cytic cells, the Be13 line is sensitive to hydrocortisone in vitro and fails to express the
natural attachment phenomena. Unlike the prothymocytes, 40% of the Be13 cells can form E rosettes. These cells also express the receptor
for the peanut agglutinin lectin PNA which is
found on the thymocytes but not on prothymo-
cythes. The Be13 line thus seems to be in an
intermediate differentiation state between pro-
thymic and thymic cells. It was of interest,
therefore, to try to induce these cells to
differentiate to a more mature state using the
phorbol ester TPA. Initial results indicate
that the Be13 cells can be partially induced to
express characteristics of a more mature differentiation state.

Department of Virology[1] and Hematology[2], Hebrew
University, Hadassah Medical School, Jerusalem,
Israel

70

PEANUT AGGLUTININ BINDING AS A DIFFERENTIATION
MARKER : ANALYSIS OF NORMAL AND MALIGNANT HUMAN
LYMPHOID CELLS
U. Galili[1], N. Galili[2] and A. Polliack[1]

The lectin peanut agglutinin (PNA) binds to D-
galactosyl and N-acetyl-galactoseamine. Agglu-
tination and fluorescence staining studies have
shown specific PNA binding to the immunoincompe-
tent cortical thymocytes. Attachment of sialic
acid to the glycoproteins during maturation of
the cortical thymocytes prevents PNA binding to
the immunocompetent T cells. It was thought that
PNA may be a marker of immature T cells and could
be used to identify malignant lymphoid cells of
T origin. This study shows that PNA binding
cannot be regarded solely as a marker for T cell
derived malignant cells. Human prothymocytes
were found to lack the PNA marker. Blood monocytes, however, exhibit strong PNA binding capacity. No correlation was found between the
differentiation stage of established T cell lines and PNA marker. Similarly, study of various
freshly isolated leukemic lymphoblastoid cells
failed to show immature T cell specificity of
the PNA marker.

1. Department of Hematology, Hadassah University
   Hospital and

2. Department of Virology, Hebrew University,
   Hadassah Medical School, Jerusalem, Israel

71

INTRA-ARTERIAL CIS-PLATINUM IN HEAD AND NECK CANCER. CON-
TROLLED CLINICAL TRIAL IN PHASES I AND II. F.C.Galmarini,
J. Yoel, J. Abulafia, J. Nakasone and G. Temperley

To evaluate response and determine the adequate administration rate and maximum tolerance dose, 33 patients with
locally advanced epidermoid carcinoma were treated with
intra-arterial Cis-platinum as per OSITC protocol 1006,
which stipulates 3 different treatment plans (A: 25 mg/m2
every 4 days; B: 40 mg/m2 every 7 days; C: 60 mg/m2 every
10 days). Nine patients were initially treated with
Scheme A, another 9 with Scheme B and 15 others with
Scheme C. Treatment duration was determined by the degree of tolerance and/or response. Maximum doses were:
Scheme A, 320 mg; B, 420 mg; C, 400 mg. Four patients
(44%) showed an objective remission over 50% with Scheme
A, 7 (77.7%) with Scheme B and 10 (66.6%) with Scheme C.
No signs of local toxicity were observed with the doses
used; this is important since it enables use before surgery and/or radiation as well as incorporation when plan-
ning polychemotherapy. It also has a low index of general toxicity. Despite a very good percentage of satisfactory responses, complete remission with histological confirmation was only observed in highly vascularized areas
(43%). Finally, analysis of results reveals that intra-
arterially administered Cis-platinum is a highly active
drug for the treatment of head and neck cancers. The
authors feel they have not yet established the optimum
dose, and thus trials are being continued with Scheme D
(75 mg/m2 every 10 days) and Scheme E (100 mg/m2 every
21 days).

Hospital Municipal de Oncologia
Patricias Argentinas 750, Buenos Aires, Argentina

72

INTRA-ARTERIAL ADRIAMYCIN IN HEAD AND NECK CANCER. F.C.
Galmarini, J. Yoel, F. Gruart, J. Nakasone, N. Peirano
Following upon R. Molinari's work, intra-arterial Adriamycin was used with highly effective results for the treatment of head and neck cancers, but this effectiveness was
partly offset by high local toxicity. Based on the pharmacokinetics of Adriamycin, a clinical trial was conducted
to establish the maximum tolerance dose at local level and
the most adequate administration rate. Of the 122 patients
treated between 1975 and 1978, 57 were put on OSITC protocol 1001 (Phase I and II study) which established 3 different dose schemes: A: 25 mg/m2 every 4 days; B: 40 mg/
m2 every 7 days; C: 60 mg/m2 every 21 days. Complete remission was found in 5 (8.8%) and remission over 50% in
22 (39%). Toxic manifestations were of both a local (stomatitis, hemifacial edema) and general nature (anemia, leukopenia) in varying degrees depending on the treatment
scheme. None of the patients developed signs of thrombocytopenia or cardiac toxicity. Based on this first trial
Adriamycin proved to be a highly valuable induction drug,
its toxicity being linked more to its rhythm of administra
tion than with the doses.
After completion of the Phase I and II study, OSITC protocol 1004 (Phase III) was undertaken with 65 evaluable patients put on 2 different dose schemes: A: 75 mg/m2 on
days 1 and 11 - 31 patients; B: 50 mg/m2 on days 1,11 and
21 - 34 patients. No significant differences were between the two schemes (Scheme A: complete remission 3%,
remission over 50%, 50%; Scheme B: complete remission 9%,
remission over 50%, 42%). As regards tolerance, Scheme B
was slightly better as concerns toxic manifestations
(stomatitis, hemifacial edema). No signs of leukopenia,
thrombocytopenia or cardiac toxicity were seen in this
patient group. We concluded that there is no evident su-
periority of one scheme over the other. Moreover, it was
confirmed that Adriamycin is an important, and posssibly
the most effective induction drug now available for intra-
arterial administration.
Hosp. Mun. de Oncologia, Buenos Aires, Argentina

73

STEM CELL ASSAY IN HUMAN BREAST CARCINOMA. D. Gangji, N. Legros, W.H.Mattheiem, M. Daniaux, B. Van den Heule and J.C. Heuson

The in vitro human tumor stem cell assay (Science, 197, 461,1977) is a potentially valuable predictive test for anticancer chemotherapy.

This system was studied in human breast cancer material. Over a 3-month period 11 primary tumor specimens (1 x 1cm) were obtained. Eight of these were processed mechanically to obtain a single cell suspension, the viability of which was poor (< 10% viable cells). Three of these preparations were cloned and did not grow. Three specimens were processed enzymatically (collagenase II and DNAase for 2 to 4 hours) and yielded a larger number of viable cells (>50%). They were successfully grown with a plating efficiency (PE) of 0.01-0.05%. Growth was inhibited by Adriamycin (10 µg/ml - 1 hr). In parallel with these preliminary trials, hormone dependance and sensitivity to cytotoxic agents were tested on two cell lines derived from human breast cancers: the MCF-7 which contains estrogen receptors (ER+) and the Evsa-T which does not (ER-). There was a linear correlation between the number of cells seeded (10^3 - 10^5 cells/dish) and the number of colonies. PE increased with the number of cells and reached a maximum at 30,000 cells/dish. PE ranged between 6 and 11% for MCF-7 and 10-30% for Evsa-T.

MCF-7 (ER+) growth was inhibited by the antiestrogen Nafoxidine (10^5 and 5.10^{-7} M) and this effect was partially reversed by estrogen (10^{-8} M). Evsa-T (ER-) was not inhibited by Nafoxidine. A panel of 14 drugs (Adm, 5-FU, VM-26, VP-16, VCR, VLB, VDS, Maytansine, PALA, Cis-DDP, Chlorozotocin, Mitomycin C, Mathyl Gag, DTIC) (10-.001 µg/ml) were tested. The pattern of sensitivity and potential for screening will be discussed.

Supported by a grant from the Fonds Cancérologique de la Caisse Générale d'Epargne et de Retraite de Belgique (CGER)

Service de Medecine, Clin. et Lab. Cancérologie Mammaire Institut Jules Bordet, Brussels, Belgium

74

AGAR BONE MARROW CULTURES: PROGNOSTIC VALUE IN ACUTE LEUKEMIA. R. Garand, M. Mouraud, E. Diez, A. and B. Le Mevel

Bone marrow (BM) granulocyte-macrophage progenitors (CFU-GM) were studied using the Pike-Robinson in vitro agar culture assay. Forty-six patients were studied at diagnosis before treatment (31 acute myeloid leukemias (AML) and 15 acute lymphoid leukemias (ALL)). Various growth patterns were observed (7th day of culture) in both types of leukemia: (1) "depletive" growth (type A) with no cluster or colony formation, or microcluster formation or weak colony formation with a normal cluster:colony ratio; and (2) "excessive" growth (type B) with macrocluster formation or colony formation. The response following chemotherapy was significantly better in AML patients with type A growth (13 complete remissions (CR) out of 19 cases (69%)) than with type B growth (2 CR out of 12 cases (16%)) (p < 0.01). This was not the case for ALL patients.

Eight AML patients were studied at relapse: 3 CRs were obtained in 5 cases of type A growth whereas the 3 type B failed to achieve CR.

47 patients (33 AML, 14 ALL) were studied during the aplastic therapeutic phase: in 17 cases no cluster or colony formation was observed, and only 2 patients entered CR (12%). In 30 patients, cultures showed various cluster/colony reformations. 19 achieved CR (70.4%) (p < 0.001).

Thus, the response to chemotherapy is significantly better in AML patients when the in vitro bone marrow growth capacity is weak before treatment. In AML and ALL, the probability of achieving CR is significantly higher in cases with CFU-GM growth reappearance.

FRA 13 - INSERM - UER Medecine Nantes, 44035 Nantes Cédex, France

75

INCIDENCE, PREVENTION AND PROGNOSIS OF SEPTICAEMIA IN PATIENTS TREATED FOR ACUTE LEUKEMIA. J.A. Gastaut, D. Maraninchi, F. Lejeune, G. Novakovitch, D. Bagarry, G. Meyer, and Y. Carcassonne

45 adult patients with A.L. received intensive aplasiant chemotherapy : 29 were in the 1st perceptible phase (P.P.) of the disease, 16 were treated in relapse. Patients were isolated in single rooms, with sterile food and total intestinal decontamination (T.I.D.).

All of them had a central catheter. Routine bacteriologic monitoring was performed weekly ; in the case of fever (≥ 38°5) blood cultures were done and a polyvalent antibiotherapy was initiated.

Of 29 patients treated in 1st P.P. 20 developed septicemia (69%) : 6 ALL (54%) and 14 AML (77%). On 16 patients treated in relapse, 12 developed septicemia (75%) : 3 ALL (50%) 9 AML (90%). The incidence of infection was very important, higher in AML than in ALL and higher in patients in relapse than in 1st P.P. Gram positive (50%) were more frequently observed than gram negative (45%) and Candida (5%). These results suggest that T.I.D. failed in this group of patients to limit infections ; an assay of Prophylactic Granulocyte Transfusion (P.G.T.)(1.4 - 0.1 x 10 ^{10}/m2/day) was done in 4 patients but 3 developed septicaemia.

In these aplastic patients the origin of infection has been rarely found (20% of the cases) ; sepsis was associated with shock in 26% of the cases ; secondary infectious foci were relatively rare. Early and intensive antibiotherapy seems to allow a good prognosis in most of the cases. Nevertheless 14 patients died of infection, among them 10 had resistant leukemia and 11 were in 2d and 3d septicemia during blastic aplasia.

The poor prognosis of infection in these patients seems linked to 3 parameters : Leukemia in relapse, blastic aplasia, multiple septicemia in the same patient. Future goals must be 1) better chemotherapy 2) better prevention (P.G.T. ? BACTRIM ? LAMINAR AIR FLOW ISOLATION ?).

INSTITUT PAOLI - CALMETTES, Service d'Hématologie 232, Bd de Sainte Marguerite - 13009 MARSEILLE.

76

PHARMACOKINETICS OF MELPHALAN IN MULTIPLE MYELOMA. E.D. Gilby and A.G. Bosanquet

Despite the widespread use of orally administered Melphalan (M) in cancer patients for 20 years, there are few reports of its pharmacokinetics in man. Recently, high pressure liquid chromatography methods have been available, and we have developed a method that will measure 5 ng/mlM. This has been used to measure serum and urine concentrations in multiple myeloma patients receiving M both orally (p.o.) and intravenously (i.v.) during normal therapy. Intravenous M decayed biphasically with half-lives of 10.2 - 2.4 min (mean - SD) and 73- 14 min. However, a large amount of the dose had disappeared from the serum even before the first (5 min) sample with an apparent volume of distribution at this time (Vd 5) of 15.2- 3.4 liters. Absorption of the drug was very variable, the area under the curve (AUC) p.o./AUC i.v. ranging from 0.29-1.14 (0.64 - 0.32). Urinary excretion of M (0-24 hr) averaged 17.0% of the dose.

Estimation of M metabolism to dihydroxy-melphalan (MOH) was made by administration of tracer tritiated M given with each dose. Counting of deproteinised serum allowed estimation of M+MOH and therefore MOH by subtraction of the HPLC result. Counting of undeproteinised serum gave figures for protein-bound radioactivity (PBM) by subtraction. AUCMOH and AUCPBM were calculated for 0-10 hr since PBM decays with a terminal half-life of approx. 7 days. In both p.o. and i.v. administration M concentrations had dropped to very low levels by 10 hours (less than 10ng/ml) and MOH accounted for only 25% of serum radioactivity. Output of tritium in urine amounted to 25.7% after p.o. and 33.3% after i.v.

The high Vd 5 found with M was also found when measuring serum tritium: this suggests there is a very rapid removal of M from the plasma in the first 5 min. This rapid removal correlates with the results of studies done with cells in tissue culture where the half-life of M uptake is about 2 min. Bioavailability of unmetabolised active M is probably greater after i.v. administration than after p.o.

Royal United Hospital, Combe Park, Bath, U.K.

20

77

ADRIAMYCIN PHARMACOKINETICS AND ABNORMAL LIVER FUNCTION
TESTS. C. Gisselbrecht, F. Lokiec, M. Marty, L. Mignot,
D. Belpomme, Y. Najean and M. Boiron.

Impairment of Adriamycin metabolism due to liver dys-
function can lead to an increase in toxicity.
In order to evaluate perturbation of Adriamycin pharmacokinetics, we studied 37 plasmatic disappearance curves
of Adriamycin in 34 patients. Dosage of Adriamycin was
determined by a radio-immunologic assay. Patients received intravenously either 35 mg/sqm or 45 mg/sqm of Adriamycin. Maximal plasmatic concentration (Cmax) ranged from
9.7. 10^{-7} M to 5.4. 10^{-5} M. No significant difference in
Cmax could be observed. In group 1, 11 control patients,
the plasmatic disappearance curve followed a triphasic
decline, with a first T 1/2 (P1) of 0.27 ± 0.19 h. the
second T 1/2 (P2) of 1.6 ± 0.9 h. and a terminal half
life of 29 ± 11 h. In group 2, 21 patients with liver
metastasis, P1 was 0.26 ± 0.15 h, P2 1.5 ± 0.9 h and P3
34 ± 20 h. No significant difference could be observed
between group 1 and group 2 although in the last group
P3 ranged from 15 h to 79 h. Total metabolic clearance
was in group 1, 53.5 ± 45 l/h-1 and $136 + 94$ l/h-1 in
group 2; the difference was not significant.
In order to see if there was a relation between liver
abnormalities and a prolonged P3 above the mean, we
looked at liver function tests in patients with P3 < 29 h
and with P3 > 29 h. Alkaline phosphatases were increased
in 7 cases on each side. K1 BSP was impaired in 5 cases
without relationship with the length of P3. Bilirubin
was abnormal only in two cases with prolonged P3 despite
a reduction dose of 1/3. No dramatic increase in hematological toxicity could be observed in patients with a
prolonged P3 except those with cirrhosis.
From these data , except for hyperbilirubinemia, liver
function tests are unable to predict abnormal Adriamycin
kinetics and reduction dose should be, at best, proposed
after pharmacokinetic study.

Hôpital Saint-Louis, Paris, France.

78

EVALUATION OF THE ASSOCIATION HEXAMETHYLMELAMINE (HMM)
ADRIAMYCIN AND PREDNISONE IN ADVANCED BREAST CANCER.
C. Gisselbrecht, L. Mignot, D. Belpomme, A. Gorins,
M. Marty, M. Boiron.

Hexamethylmelamine (HMM) is a triazine derivative which
may function as an antimetabolite although it was initially thought to be an alkylating agent. In early
broad phase II trials, response rates of 13% - 23% were
reported in breast carcinoma. The present trial was
undertaken to determine the response to the not yet
tested association of HMM - Adriamycin - Prednisone in
metastatic breast cancer. 20 patients (mean age: 54 y.)
were treated every month with HMM 6mg/kg/d per os from
d. 1 to d. 15, adriamycin 30mg/m2 intravenously on d. 1
and d. 8, prednisone 0.75mg/kg/d for fifteen days.
3 patients had received previously C.M.F. chemotherapy.
All patients received at least one cycle (m = 3.3.,
range: 1 to 8).
Response rate was: C.R.complete response 20%, partial
response 30%, stable 30%, failure 20%. The duration of
response was 5 months for responders.
Gastrointestinal toxicity was mild in 40% and severe in
25% of the patients. Reduction dose of HMM was necessary in 50%. Mild neutropenia was observed in 25%. Neurotoxicity was present in 20% with numbness in 10%.
The response rate of 50% obtained with HMM-Adriamycin is
comparable to other chemotherapy combinations used in
breast cancer. The lack of hematotoxicity allows ambulatory treatment. However, because of gastrointestinal
toxicity this association can not be recommended for
routine treatment.
Supported by N.C.I.-French American cancer research
agreement.

Hôpital Saint Louis, Paris, France

79

PRESENCE OF VARIOUS SURFACE MARKERS ON THE MEM-
BRANES OF LEUKEMIA AND LYMPHOMA CELL LINES AND
CELL HYBRIDS
N.Goldblum[2], S.Mitrani[2], C.Billard[1], M.C.Martyré[1],
M.Kayibanda[1], Z.Mishal[1], T.Hercend[1], A.Goutner[1],
R.Ber[3], C.Boucheix[1] and C. Rosenfeld[1]

Several human leukemia and lymphoma cell lines
were studied for the presence of CALLA antigen.
In addition to an absorbed rabbit heteroanti-
serum to CALLA, a "more specific" monoclonal
antibody (J-5,Ritz et al. Nature,283,583-585,
1980)was used.Certain cell lines were found
equally reactive with both CALLA and J-5 (Daudi
and Reh). Other cell lines, such as DG-75, a non
EBV genome carrying Burkitt lymphoma line and
HD-Mar, a T-cell leukemia cell, were highly reactive (up to 100% of the cells) with CALLA but
were either completely(DG-75)or partially(HD-Mar)
negative with J-5. A hybrid cell line, Hu/Dut,
prepared by fusing of Daudi with a human epithelial cell line U, reacted neither with CALLA nor
with J-5, indicating that the expression of
the   glycoprotein(s) on the surface membrane
is completely inhibited in this hybrid. IgM and
Kappa as well as Ia which are present on the
surface of all parent Daudi cells were also completely absent in the hybrid. Hu/Dut carries,
however, EBV genome(s), as indicated by a highly
positive reaction for the intranuclear EBNA
antigen.
This work was supported by grants from CNAMTS,
DGRST(80.7.226),UER Kremlin Bicêtre(782) and
INSERM (82.79.114)
1.Dept.Cult. et Prod. Cell. Humaines, I.C.I.G.
  INSERM U.50, Villejuif, France
2.Dept. of Virology, Hadassah Medical School,
  Hebrew University, Jerusalem , Israel
3.Technion Medical School, Haifa, Israel

80

THE LONG TERM OUTLOOK FOR CHILDREN TREATED FOR NON-
HODGKIN'S LYMPHOMA. A.J.Goldman

29 children with non-Hodgkin's lymphomas were treated,
between 1974 and 1977, with a protocol designed by the
Royal Marsden/St.Bartholomew's Hospitals'Children's
Solid Tumour Group (CSTG). 79% had advanced disease and
all had Rappaport's diffuse histology. The protocol involved induction, cranial prophylaxis and a three drug maintenance scheme with multiple drug intensification every
8 weeks, for 3 years. 18 patients (62%) achieved a complete remission. 12 patients (41%) remain alive and disease-free at this time. 8 patients have relapsed; 2 in
the C.N.S. who are both in second remissions and off all
therapy, 5 in the bone marrow, 2 in the testes and 1 in
the mediastinum who have died. Comparison with a historical control group of 23 patients shows a significant
improvement in survival   (p= .005) 22 of the controls
have died.
The protocol proved moderately toxic, particularly to
the bone marrow, necessitating modification in the length
and intensity of maintenance in some patients. There were
no treatment-related deaths.
The results confirm that the outlook for children with
non-Hodgkin's lymphoma can be greatly improved by regarding the disease as disseminated at diagnosis and using
cranial prophylaxis and intensive multiple drug regimens.
It has encouraged the development of further protocols
incorporating a wider variety of active drugs.

A report of the Children's Solid Tumour Group, Royal
Marsden Hospital, and St.Bartholomew's Hospital,
London, England

81

M-AMSA (4 (9-ACRIDINYLAMINO) METHANESULPHON-M-
ANISIDINE) IN CHILDREN WITH WIDESPREAD MALIGNANT DISEASE.

A.J. Goldman, F.L. Dudley, J.S. Malpas

AMSA has been given to 11 children using two schedules.
Five children with haematological malignancies received
doses from $25mg/m^2$ daily for 3 days escalating to $150mg/m^2$
for 5 days. Six children with solid tumours received
single doses from $120mg/m^2$ escalating to $180mg/m^2$. The
drug was diluted in 5% dextrose and infused over two
hours and courses were repeated 3 weekly. All patients
were heavily pretreated.

Myelosuppression, in particular leukopaenia, always
occurred but was only a limiting factor at the highest
doses. Thrombocytopaenia was seen at the higher dose
levels. Other side effects were mild nausea, vomiting,
phlebitis, general malaise, mucositis and pain at the
site of metastases during drug administration.

No complete responses were seen. One patient with
haematological disease achieved a markedly hypoplastic
marrow with disappearance of blast cells after a total
dose of $500mg/m^2$ but he refused further therapy and this
remission was short. Three children had temporary
reductions in their peripheral blast counts. No
significant responses have been seen so far with solid
tumours. The growth of multiple secondaries from a
retinoblastoma appeared to be delayed over 3 courses
of AMSA. Some activity of AMSA has been demonstrated
which warrants further investigation.

Royal Marsden Hospital, Fulham Road, London, U.K.

83

PHARMACOKINETICS OF CYCLOPHOSPHAMIDE IN CANCER PATIENTS.
B. Gourmel, C. Gisselbrecht, M. Marty, R. Julien,
D. Blais, C. Dreux, M. Boiron

Although cyclophosphamide (CPA) is one of the most widely
used anticancer agents, pharmacological studies in man
have not been extensive, apart from those using radio-
labelled drug. We have developed such studies using gas-
liquid chromatography with a salt detector (NPSD). The
parent drug as well as iphosphamide (internal standard)
diluted in plasma samples were submitted to ethyl-acetate
extraction followed by evaporation and fluoration
(70° C for 20 min). Derivatives were then injected onto
an OV 17 (3%) column. Internal and CPA standards were
prepared by dilution in each patient's plasma obtained
before CPA infusion. This method allows quantitation of
plasma CPA concentrations over 20 ng/ml with excellent
specificity (r=0.99).
CPA pharmacokinetics were performed in 11 pts treated
with CPA (750 to 2200 mg/sqm) given as a 1-hr infusion.
All except two had normal renal and liver function tests.
Peak plasma levels were achieved at the end of the infusion and ranged from 38.6 µg/ml to 99.7 µg/ml. Although
the number of pts is still small, there appears to be few
individual variations in the peak plasma levels (15%).
Plasma disappearance follows a biexponential pattern.
However, individual variations are considerable as the
first half-life ranged from 30 to 60 min while the terminal half-life ranged from 210 to 610 minutes. This method
allows rapid, sensitive and specific determinations of
unchanged plasma CPA levels. As dosage can be performed
with 100 µl plasma samples, simultaneous study of other
anticancer drugs can easily be performed. However, detection of CPA metabolites using the same procedures lacks
specificity as some metabolites (4OHCPA) undergo degrada-
tion during experimental steps.

Groupe de Pharmacologie Clinique des Anticancéreux
Hôpital St Louis, 2 place du Dr Fournier, 75010 Paris

Supported by INSERM (French-American agreement)

82

FUNCTIONAL KINETIC STUDY OF STRONTIUM 85 FOR ONE HUNDRED
OSTEOGENIC SARCOMAS. R. Gongora, A. Mazabraud, G. Gongora
B. Perdereau

For the past 10 years we have been carrying out a functional kinetic study of 85 Sr, whose metabolism, as is
well known, is almost the same as that of calcium. The
procedure involves intravenous injection of 50 micro-
curies of 85 Sr chloride which enables external measurement over a period of 8 days. Measurements are made on a
daily basis on both the tumoral and the symmetric region,
which serves as a reference. Results of this test are expressed as the ratio between the tumoral zone and the
healthy symmetric bone region. This test has shown that
osteogenic sarcomas can be broken down into 3 distinct
groups, defined by the ratio value on the last day of
testing (R8) and, for instance, by R8-R1, representing
the average gradient between the 1st and 8th days of
testing. The mathematical expression of the curves is
logarithmic for the 3 groups, according to the formula:
y=a+bln x. Incomparing histological sections of the sarcomas with the results of this test, we noted that osteogenic sarcomas with a descending curve (type 1) include
anaplastic sarcomas (which appear to be very lytic on
X-rays), most of the telangiectatic sarcomas, plus a certain number of slightly osteogenic sarcomas. The prognosis
for these tumors is very poor. Sarcomas with ascending
curves (types 2 and 3) are obviously osteogenic and have
a better prognosis. This functional kinetic test seemed
to us to be of prognostic value. Moreover, it allows
assessment of therapeutic results if repeated. Kinetic
functional studies of 85 Sr were also conducted for bone
lymphomas and Ewing's sarcomas, which have quite different curves.

Institut Curie
26 rue d'Ulm
75231 Paris Cédex 05, France

84

IN VIVO AND IN VITRO MODULATION OF NATURAL
KILLER CELL ACTIVITY
A. Goutner, J.L. Misset, P. Ribaud and G. Mathé

Natural killer cells (NK) are a subpopulation of
mononuclear cells that are cytotoxic to varie-
ties of malignant cells and could be responsible
for an in vivo antitumour effect. We have studied the effect of leucocytic interferon in
chronic lymphoid leukaemia patients, of fibroblastic interferon in myeloma patients and of a
lymphokine preparation in breast cancer patients,
on their NK cell activity measured in vitro in a
51chromium release assay using K562 target cells.

In vivo NK cell activity can be enhanced four to
sixteen fold by leucocytic and fibroblastic
interferons and by a preparation of lymphokines
devoided of interferon. The stimulation of NK
cells disappears after high doses or prolonged
administration of interferon. If NK cells are
responsible for the therapeutic effects of these
biological mediators, this stresses the importance
of the immunological monitoring.

In vitro NPT 15392, a new synthetic immunomodu-
lator which is a derivative of isoprinosine,
is able to augment NK cell activity and to
enhance the stimulatory effect of interferon.
Prostaglandin E at $10^{-7}M$ can suppress in vitro
the cytotoxic potential of NK cells. Thus various mediators and synthetic molecules can
regulate negatively or positively the cytotoxicity of NK cells.

Hôpital Paul-Brousse : Institut de Cancérologie
et d'Immunogénétique (INSERM U-50), 94800-
Villejuif, France.

22

85

PREVENTION OF DRUG-INDUCED ALOPECIA IN CANCER PATIENTS.
M. Grandjean, D. Belpomme, E. Pujade-Lauraine, M. Marty,
M. Boiron

The preventive effect of local hypothermia against drug-
induced alopecia (J.C.Dean et al., N.Eng. J. Med., 301,
1427, 1979), was studied in 33 cancer patients receiving
different combinations of chemotherapy and compared to a
control group of 36 patients previously treated with comparable drug combinations without local hypothermia.
Hypothermia consisted of ice packing of the scalp 15 min.
before, during and 15 min. after IV administration of
chemotherapy.
In the hypothermia group, 60.3% of patients did not experience alopecia; furthermore, some of them had hair
regrowth during chemotherapy (evolution A), 21.5% had
slight alopecia (evolution B) and 17.2% considerable
alopecia necessitating a wig (evolution C).
In the control group, A was found in 28.8%, B in 11.4%
and C in 59.8% of cases. Although evolution of A, B and
C were similar with reference to the type of chemotherapy, alopecia was nonetheless most important with regimens
including Doxorubycin and Cyclophosphamide.
This data strongly suggests that local hypothermia is a
powerful means of avoiding alopecia when chemotherapy is
administered by short IV courses.

Département de Cancérologie
Hôpital Saint Louis, Paris

86

AN ATTEMPT AT XENOGENEIC IMMUNE RNA MEDIATED TRANSFER OF
IMMUNITY TO SOLUBLE BLAST CELL EXTRACTS IN VITRO. O.Guerci
B.Weber, J.Pierrez, C.Janot, F.Schooneman, D.Oth, O.Belotti
E.Marbache.
We conducted a lymphoblastic transformation assay with iso-
topic labelling by micromethod to demonstrate that normal
non-immune human peripheral blood lymphocytes are converted
into immune lymphocytes against soluble extract from blast
cells by xenogeneic immune RNA.
-RNA is obtained from the lymph nodes and spleen of a sheep
immunized with blast cells mixed with BCG and CFA. We extracted RNA with hot phenol and with ether. Then RNA rich
extract is precipitated with ethanol and NaCl. The conser-
vative procedure is lyophilisation at 4°C. RNA concentration is estimated by the orcinol reaction; DNA by dipheny-
lamine reaction and protein by the Lowry method. Ultracen-
trifugation of RNA preparation with U.V.scanner using a
band sedimentation technique (on 1M NaCl 20°C) pointed out
5S and 18S RNA components in all samples and often 10-13S
component.
-Peripheral blood lymphocytes from healthy donors are incubated with I RNA, then washed and grown in presence of soluble blast cell extract (prepared according to MAVLIGIT's
method). The lymphocyte : blast cell extract ratio was
10^5 : 0.1 to 0.5 µg of antigeneic protein. TH_3 incorporation rate by these lymphocytes was compared with that
of RNA untreated lymphocytes. Controls consisted of : RNA
treated and RNA untreated lymphocytes alone and in presence of PHA.
The results show : RNA does not improve the spontaneous incorporation rate of TH_3 by lymphocytes, nor in presence of
PHA; when increasing soluble blast cell extract protein
concentration the TH_3 incorporation decreases; in presence
of low concentration of blast cell **extract** TH_3 incorporation by lymphocytes is significantly improved by the lymphocytes that have been incubated before with RNA rich extract containing 10-13 component. These experiences suggest
that RNA 10-13 component could transfer immunity against
blast cell extract.
Serv.Med.Générale,Maison Hosp.StCharles, 54 NANCY, France

87

LATE RESULTS IN TREATEENT OF TESTICULAR NEOPLASMS J.Guerrin
P. Fargeot, C. de Gislain. L. Boyer.

In recent years numerous studies have shown a real improvement in the prognosis of testicular tumors by the use of chemotherapy. In 1975 at the ffrst congress of the European Society for Medical Oncology the authors reported three observations of advanced testicular tumors whose follow-up was 23,28
and 48 months respectively. Complete remission was obtained
following chemotherapy. Hope of total cure is allowed and most
investigators believe that a new evolution of these tumors
over three years after diagnosis is exceptional.
Our present work is concerned with the late outlook of patients treated for malignant testicular tumors. It reviews
125 patients seen from 1966 to 1977 at the cancer institute
of Dijon (Centre Georges-François Leclerc). Of these patients,
79 have non-seminomatous germinal cell tumors, 39 seminomas
and 7 lymphomas. Forty-four deaths happened during the first
three-year follow-up : 34 among non seminomatous germinal
cell tumors, 5 in seminomas and 5 also in lymphomas. Two patients with seminomas and 2 with non seminomatous germinal
cell tumors died later : 2 of them had an intercurrent cardio-
vascular disease, a third one had squamous cell carcinoma
localised both at the oral cavity and at the oesophagus and
a fourth one had epidural and pulmonary metastatic evolution
of his seminoma as long as seven years after diagnosis.
Forty-five cases of non seminomatous germinal cell tumors
were free of disease at the third year of follow up. Disease
recurrence came in 3 during the fourth year of follow up and
in one during the seventh year. Three cases demonstrated pulmonary metastases at the time of diagnosis : 2 relapsed at
this site and the third one presented rather an inguinal
lymph node involvement ; the other one revealed pulmonary
spreading at the time of relapse only. A special attention is
given to clinical presentation, pathological documents and
therapeutic approach of these patients.
Finally, unexpected problems which patients cured over three
years of diagnosis have to face   are analysed.

Centre Georges-Francois Leclerc, rue du Pr Marion, Dijon.

88

AN ACUTE LYMPHOBLASTIC LEUKAEMIA ASSOCIATED ANTIGEN.
C. Guibout, J.F. Doré[+] and E. Archimbaud.[+]

An antiserum was raised in a monkey against fresh cells
from a patient with non T, non B acute lymphoblastic leukaemia (ALL) and absorbed against pooled human red blood
cells and cells from a B lymphoblastoid cell line established by in vitro infection of the patient's lymphocytes with EBV. The reactivity pattern of this antiserum
was studied in a microcytotoxicity assay using cells
from 23 lines established from normal blood or various
leukaemias and lymphomas. The absorbed antiserum reacts
with 1/2 T-ALL lines (Molt-4), 1 B-ALL line, 4/4 non T,
non B-ALL lines, 0/2 myeloid lines, 1/3 Burkitt lymphoma lines,(Daudi),1/10 B lymphoblastoïd cell lines of normal or leukaemic origin, and does not react with an endometrial carcinoma line expressing Ia-like antigen. Further absorption of the antiserum with Molt-4 cells abolished its reactivity with Molt-4 and Daudi lines without
modifying its reactivity with B or non T, non B-ALL
lines. Absorption of the antiserum with Daudi cells,
which are known to express both the Daudi and the cALL
differentiation antigens, abolished its reactivity with
Daudi and a non T, non B-ALL line (KM-3), but did not
modify its reactivity with the other ALL lines.

This antiserum is likely to detect an acute lymphoblastic leukaemia associated antigen serologically different
from the previously identified Daudi and cALL antigens.

[+]Institut de Cancérologie et d'Immunogénétique, 94800
Villejuif, and[+]INSERM FRA 24, Centre Léon Bérard,
69373 Lyon Cédex 2, France.

89

MULTIPLE BIOCHEMICAL MARKERS IN FOLLOW-UP OF OVARIAN CANCER, W.G.Haije, E.H.Cooper, S.Haworth, J.Meerwaldt & A.Roberts

In 31 patients treated for ovarian cancer and followed for >2 years a battery of biochemical markers were evaluated. They included: Phosphohexose isomerase (PHI), C-reactive protein (CRP), α_1 Acid Glycoprotein, Albumin (ALB), Pre-albumin (PAB), Transferrin (TSF), β2-Microglobulin (32-m), Sex hormone binding globulin, Carcinoembryonic antigen (CEA) and Placental-like Alkaline Phosphatase (PAP).

In 10 patients who had no evidence of disease during follow-up, the markers stayed almost without exception within normal limits with only minor fluctuations. In some patients raised CEA was found. Of 5 patients with tumours who responded favourably to therapy, some markers were raised when tumour was present (PAP 5x, PHI 2x, CRP 1x) and returned to normal afterwards. CFA showed less consistent values. The other markers had normal values.
16 patients did not respond to therapy: the tumours tended to progress or there were recurrences. 12 of them died during follow-up.
In this group of badly controlled patients, many biochemical disturbances were found: PAP & CEA were often raised, sometimes progressivoly; PHI & β2-m values in many patients fluctuated above the normal level. In most cases a significant drop in ALB values (accompanied by declining PAB & TSF concentrations) was seen together with a marked rise of CRP levels.

Longitudinal studies of some of these markers have potential as an aid to contribute to the management of patients with ovarian cancer.

Rotterdamsch Radio-Therapeutisch Instituut. Rotterdam.

90

DETECTION OF HYALURONECTIN OR MESENCHYME ASSOCIATED ANTIGEN IN THE EARLY STAGES OF COLONIC CARCINOGENESIS WITH 1,2-DIMETHYLHYDRAZINE. E.Halkin, B.Delpech, R.Laumonier

This study dealt with the detection of a protein "hyaluronectin" in the colon of DMH intoxicated rats. Hyaluronectin is a hyaluronic binding glycoprotein that is associated with foetal, reactive or cancerous mesenchyme. Immunochemistry study used the indirect method with an immunserum conjugated with peroxidase. The dose dependence, the latency period of hyaluronectin production in tumours and preneoplastic lesions induced by DMH treatment have been demonstrated in the present work. These observations establish two points of conclusion :
1) a correlation exists between carcinogenesis and hyaluronectin accumulation;
2) the dose dependence and evolution of the process suggests that the content of colonic mucosa is related to the content of "pretransformed cells".
Hyaluronectin or mesenchyme associated antigen could be considered a marker of the initiation stage of carcinogenesis.

Centre Henri Becquerel, Department of Experimental Cancerology and Pathology, 76038 Rouen, France

91

AMINOGLUTETHIMIDE IN ADVANCED BREAST CANCER:CORRELATION OF OESTROGEN SUPPRESSION WITH RESPONSE.A.L.Harris,M.Dowsett, S.L.Jeffcoate,I.E.Smith.
Aminoglutethimide (AG) with glucocorticoid replacement achieves a response (R) in over 30% of patients with advanced breast cancer[1],[2]. AG inhibits both adrenal steroid synthesis (medical adrenalectomy) and peripheral aromatase[2]. Some patients whose tumours are positive for oestrogen receptors fail to respond, and inadequate oestrogen suppression may be a reason for failure. We have measured hormone profiles after a mean of 3 months treatment with AG. So far 20 patients have progressive disease (PD) (median± age 53 years, disease free interval 1 year, years post-menopausal 10 years), and 14 have achieved an objective response (R) (median±age 56 years, disease free interval 2.25 years, years post-menopausal 10 years), as assessed by standard UICC criteria.
Oestrone, the main oestrogen in post-menopausal women was significantly lower in R than in PD (R 168+77 pmol/l, PD 303+108 pmol/l, P <0.01 Wilcoxon ranked sums). Sex hormone binding globulin (SHBG) was significantly lower in R (44.3+ 16.9) than in PD (68.2+25, P <0.01). This probably reflects the less oestrogenic environment in R. No significant difference was found in dehydroepiandrosterone sulphate (DHA-S), the best monitor of adrenal suppression, nor in 17 OH progesterone,androstenedione, testosterone, oestradiol, prolactin, FSH, or LH (all measured by radio-immunoassay). These results suggest that peripheral aromatase inhibition by AG may be more important than its adrenal suppression effect. It is possible that increasing doses of AG may produce further inhibition of aromatase, and oestrone could be monitored in non-responders.
[1]Smith et al, Lancet 2:646 1978.
[2]Lawrence et al., Cancer 45: 786 1980.

Royal Marsden Hospital, Fulham Road, London, SW3.
Chelsea Hospital For Women, Dove House Street, London,SW3.

92

AMINOGLUTETHIMIDE IN PREMENOPAUSAL WOMEN WITH BREAST CANCER:ENDOCRINE STUDIES AND TUMOUR RESPONSE.A.L.Harris, M.Dowsett,I.E.Smith,S.L.Jeffcoate,M.Morgan,J.A.McKinna.
Aminoglutethimide (AG) with glucocorticoid replacement (medical adrenalectomy) achieves a 30% response rate in advanced breast cancer in post-menopausal women. It has also been reported to reduce ovarian oestrogen production by 50% in normal premenopausal women (Corhery et al. AACR 944, 1979). We have treated 16 premenopausal patients with breast cancer, 12 with advanced disease, 4 as adjuvant therapy. Hormone profiles were measured before starting treatment and 2-4 weekly afterwards. In 3 patients ovarian response to Pergonal was measured before and 1 month after AG.
In 3 patients there was prolonged irregular menstruation and 3 patients had less heavy periods. 10/12 patients with advanced disease were assessable for tumour response. 9 had progressive disease and one had subjective response or bone pain.
Oestrone, oestradiol, sex hormone binding globulin, dehydroepiandrosterone sulphate (DHAS), 17 OH progesterone, FSH, LH and prolactin were measured. In only one patient was there suppression of oestradiol below the normal range. None had levels in the range of oophorectomised patients. In 3 patients assessed for ovarian response to Pergonal there was no suppression in 2 patients, and suppression in 1. However DHAS, a measure of adrenal suppression, was depressed in all patients into the range found in post-menopausal patients. AG cannot therefore be used alone in premenopausal patients but could be combined with oestrogen receptor blockers or oophorectomy.

Royal Marsden Hospital, Fulham Road, London, SW3.
Chelsea Hospital For Women, Dove House Street, London,SW3.

93

ACUTE ADULT MYELOGENOUS LEUKAEMIA: A RANDOMISED TRIAL OF IMMUNOTHERAPY COMPARED WITH NO MAINTENANCE TREATMENT
R. Harris, A.P. Read, S.R. Zuhrie, C.B. Freeman and I.W. Delamore.

This trial compared the effects of active immunotherapy uncomplicated by maintenance chemotherapy with randomised controls who received neither immunotherapy nor maintenance chemotherapy. Remission was induced by Daunorubesin and Cytosine Arabinoside followed by six weeks consolidation therapy with cyclophosphamide plus 6-Thioguanine. Of 41 patients, 21 were randomised to immunotherapy consisting of intradermal BCG plus allogeneic leukaemic cells and 20 were randomised to "no maintenance". Prospective ABO, Rh and HLA typing was performed before treatment was commenced. Using the Log Rank test patients receiving immunotherapy had significantly longer remission and survival from remission. Our previous observations on the effects of survival genes in AML were consistent with a differential response to immunotherapy. Providing adequate consolidation chemotherapy has been used, active immunotherapy prolongs first remission and survival from remission to a modest but statistically significant extent and clearly indicates the need for further study of the underlying biological phenomena.

Departments of Medical Genetics and Clinical Haematology, Central District, Manchester, England.

94

THYMIDINE UPTAKE BY BLOOD AND BONE MARROW CELLS IN CHRONIC MYELOCYTIC LEUKEMIA(CML). R.Herrmann, G.A. Gomez, C. Darlak, J.E. Sokal

^{3}H-thymidine (^{3}H-TdR) uptake by blood and marrow cells was determined simultaneously by the whole blood method in 70 pts. with CML, followed for up to 3 1/2 years. At each determination, pts. were classified into one of 4 phases: 1) chronic controlled (WBC<10,000, Hct>30%, platelets >100,000, marrow blasts<5%); 2) chronic uncontr. (WBC>10,000, circulating blasts<4%); 3) accelerated (Hct<30% or platel.<100,000 or increased blasts/promyelocytes(PMC) or treatment resistant splenomegaly or myeloblastomas or major karyotypic change); 4) blastic (circulating blasts+PMC >30% or marrow blasts>20%). The mean ^{3}H-TdR uptake (DPM/10^{3}WBC) was lower in phase 1 (5.5)than in phase 2 (16, p<0.001), phase 3 (24, p<0.001) and phase 4 (36, p<0.001). ^{3}H-TdR uptake in marrow was highest in phase 1 (113) and lower in phase 2 (58, p<0.001), phase 3 (83, p<0.05) and phase 4 (73, p<0.01). The difference between phase 2 and phase 4 was most prominent in the blood uptake (p<0.001); between phase 3 and phase 4 it was most prominent in the ratio of marrow and blood uptake (8.1 vs 2.2, p<0.001). These results show that the different clinical phases of CML are characterized by a different ^{3}H-TdR uptake pattern. More frequent determinations of ^{3}H-TdR uptake in the peripheral blood might provide early warning of progression to a terminal phase of CML.

Dr. Richard Herrmann
Medizinische Universitätsklinik
D-6900 Heidelberg   West Germany

95

NON-HODGKIN'S LYMPHOMAS (NHL) - TREATMENT OF LOCALIZED RELAPSES WITH CHEMO+ BCG-THERAPY.
B. Hœrni, M. Durand, P. Richaud, H. Eghbali, G. Hœrni-Simon

The usefulness of maintenance BCG (I) in the treatment of NHL, mainly in clinical stages I and II after chemo (C) - and radio (R) therapy has been previously demonstrated by a randomized trial (Br J Haematol 1979 ; 42 : 507-14). The results were particularly significant for patients treated after an initial relapse : there were only 2 relapses out of 12 BCG-treated patients vs. 10/14 controls (p = 0.0052). We present here all patients in relapse treated with C-R-C-I in a prospective controlled trial from July 1974 to April 1980.
Twenty-two patients, 12 males and 10 females, were in first (14) second (5) or further (3) relapse ; their median age was 51 y (range : 35-77). Histology, according to Kiel's classification, was low grade for 18 and high grade for 4 patients. The median delay from diagnosis to considered relapse was 33 mo. (7-135). All patients had previously received radiotherapy and 14 also received chemotherapy. After a clinical-radiologic work up, 9 patients were classified as clinical stage I ; 8 as stage II, 2 as stage III and 3 as stage IV. All patients were put into complete remission by chemoradiotherapy. They then received one course of reinforcement chemotherapy and lastly BCG by weekly skin scarifications. The median follow-up is 23 mo. Only three patients relapsed again after 2, 4 and 6 mo ; there were no relapses between 6 and 60 mo for 16 patients. Thus, it seems possible to cure a high proportion of patients with NHL in relapse provided the disease is not too largely disseminated at that time, mainly in low grade malignancy (only one relapse out of 18 patients). More patients and longer follow-up are required to clarify these results.

Fondation Bergonié, 180 rue de Saint Genès, F33076 Bordeaux Cédex

96

A NEW FIRST LINE REGIME FOR ADVANCED BREAST CANCER. HIGH DOSE CYTOXAN. HIGH DOSE 5 F-U. L. Israel, J.L. Breau

25   consecutive patients evaluable in July 1980 have yielded a 100 % response rate with a combination of CTX 1.250 g/m^2 day 1 and FU 600 mg/m^2 day 1 to 5, every 3 weeks. 8 patients had inflammatory carcinomas and underwent mastectomy after 2 to 3 cycles. All were put in > 50% partial regression. All are disease free between 6+ and 18+ months after operation, under the same regime with dose descalation. 17 patients had visceral metastases. 8 experienced a complete response, maintained between 5+ and 20+ months. CR may appear until the 10th course. 9 have had so far > 50 % partial responses, maintained between 5+ and 19+ months, except for one who relapsed at 18 months under treatment and another who stopped the therapy at 18 months and had a recurrence later. Some of these partial responses have already reached 80 % to 90 % and are expected to be put into a state of CR.

Toxicity   is moderate to high with WBL below 1000 in most cases, necessitating afterwards a dose descalation of 20 %. No drug related death has been observed. These highly encouraging results, obtained with two drugs at the maximum tolerated dose will be explained in terms of pharmacokinetics. They seem to indicate :

1) that clinical resistance should not be equated to in vitro resistance, which has been probably overestimated ;

2) that as long as toxicity is tolerable, cytostatic drugs should be employed in a continuous fashion.

They warrant further studies with fewer drugs at higher doses as opposed to conventional regimes.

CHU Bobigny, 93000 France

97

CORRELATION BETWEEN LYMPH NODE STATUS AND PREOPERATIVE MACROPHAGE CHEMOTAXIS. A SINGLE HIGHLY PREDICTIVE TEST FOR MONITORING IMMUNE STATUS. L. Israel, R. Samak, D. Bogucki, M. Samak

Absolute numbers of macrophages migrating between 12 and 24 hours towards a skin abrasion area have been counted in 107 preoperative patients (75 bronchial carcinomas, 30 breast cancers, 2 GI cancers). Findings are as follows:
(1) 65 patients later found to have positive nodes had macrophage numbers significantly below controls.
(2) Of these 65, 8 patients nevertheless had numbers over those of the controls and had only one positive node.
(3) 42 patients with negative nodes were significantly higher than controls, showing an ability to be stimulated by an early, localized tumor.
(4) However, 8 of these 42 patients had numbers significantly below those of the controls, and 3 were found to have metastases within 6 months.

The test described here accurately evaluates the biological situation reflected in the lymph node status and the spread of the disease. It should be done routinely in presurgical patients and could also serve as a marker for assessing the effectiveness of biological response modifiers.
This test, which explores the nonspecific chemotaxis of macrophages in vivo, is, is our experience, more accurate than any other in vivo or in vitro test in predicting lymph node status. The implications of the overstimulated state of negative node patients will be discussed.

CHU Bobigny, 93000 France

98

ADJUVANT CHEMOTHERAPY IN COLORECTAL CARCINOMA.
Cl. Jacquillat, G. Auclerc, M. Weil, M.F. Auclerc

Adjuvant chemotherapy in colorectal carcinoma (Dukes' stage B2 and C) does not appear to significantly increase the survival of patients. However, all randomized studies with 5-Fluorouracil (5-FU) alone or combined with methyl CCNU (MeCCNU) showed best results with chemotherapy even if none has been positive. However, Higgins recently found no difference in the five-year survival between a control group and patients treated by 5-FU alone or 5-FU plus MeCCNU. It thus seems that adjuvant 5-FU must be associated with other active drugs to improve the prognosis. This is why, in 1977, we initiated a multicentric randomized study of Dukes' A,B and C colorectal carcinoma. There were two treatment groups: 5-FU (350 mg/m2/day for 5 days every week) versus Vinblastine + Thiotepa + Methotrexate + 5-FU (VTMF, 1 course every 4 weeks) during 6 months for Dukes' A and 12 months for Dukes' B and C. Of 125 randomized patients, 113 were eligible. Fifteen relapses were observed (7 Dukes' C): 7 of them in the 5-FU group (52 patients) and 8 in the VTMF group (61 patients). Four year survival without evidence of disease is 85% overall in both groups: 90% in the 5-FU group and 70% in the VTMF group. These results seem better than those observed in historical controls, but no difference appears between the two treatments at this time. After curative resection, we now compare, in Dukes' A, abstention and 5-FU + hydroxyurea (HU) for 6 months, and in Dukes' B and C, 5-FU + HU versus 5-FU + Adriamycin + Mitomycin C (FAM) every month for one year.

Unité de Chimiothérapie, Hôpital St Louis
2 place du Dr Fournier
75475 Paris Cédex 10, France

99

ACUTE LYMPHOBLASTIC LEUKEMIA - PROTOCOL 08 LA 74
Cl. Jacquillat, M.F. Auclerc, M. Weil, G. Auclerc

In 1973, the retrospective analysis of 559 children showed three distinct prognostic classes when the same treatment was applied to all children. The objectives were (1) to test the significance of addition of Cyclophosphamide (CTX) to the combination Prednisone + Vincristine + Daunorubicine to eliminate the prognostic handicaps by adjustment of doses; (2) to compare in patients who underwent prophylactic cranial irradiation the value of I.T. Methotrexate + Ara-C + Methyl-Prednisolone to Methotrexate + Methyl-Prednisolone and (3) to compare the advantages of prolongation or discontinuation of treatment after 3, 4 and 5 years depending on the prognostic class.
403 children less than 20 years of age entered this protocol. FAB classification was applied to 123 children from Saint Louis Hospital. The percentage of remission is the same (90%) whether the treatment includes CTX or not, except for the poor prognosis group (class 3). However, there is a non-significant advantage. The main factors influencing the rate of complete remission are sex, age, WBC (35,000/mm3), platelets (100,000/mm3), and tumors (spleen, liver, lymph nodes). All of these parameters also influence the duration of remission (except age). The five-year survival without any relapse is 44%: no difference is observed with or without CTX. Prognostic stratification based on the addition of the parameters does not consider their interaction. We therefore applied Cox's method to our analysis for better discrimination and observed many discrepancies.

Unité de Chimiothérapie, Hôpital St Louis
2 place du Dr Fournier
75475 Paris Cédex 10, France

100

POOR PROGNOSIS ACUTE LYMPHOBLASTIC LEUKEMIA.
Cl. Jacquillat, M. Weil, M.F. Auclerc, G. Schaison, G. Auclerc

Burkitt's type leukemias have specific cytologic, immunologic and cytogenetic characteristics. Initial symptomatology frequently includes abdominal tumors and initial CNS involvement. Despite intensive treatment, including high dose Cyclophosphamide, prognosis remains poor in most patients (pts) because of failures to achieve active complete remission or because of early relapses (especially CNS relapses). Class III child ALL is defined by the presence of two or more unfavorable parameters (age $\geq$ 15 yr; WBC $\geq$ 35,000; spleen or liver enlargement $\geq$ 6 cm; or lymph node enlargement $\geq$ 3 cm).
Class III pts have a median duration of complete remission of less than 12 months, and less than 25% are in complete remission at 2 years. Recent progress has been achieved by intensive therapy. Cox's multifactorial analysis allows improved discrimination. We have thus defined as very increased risk ALL (VIRCALL) pts with T markers and/or pts with thymic enlargement. Pts in these categories before 1974 had a complete remission at one year rate of 21% and 23%. A phase I protocol for VIRCALL, including preventative testis irradiation and monthly reinductions without continuous maintenance for the first six months of complete remission, seems promising.

Unité de Chimiothérapie, Hôpital St Louis
2 place du Dr Fournier
75475 Paris Cédex 10, France

101

EFFECTS OF RADIOTHERAPY ON THE STEROID RECEPTOR LEVELS IN
HUMAN BREAST CARCINOMA. J.Ph.Janssens, J.Bonte,
A.Drochmans, J.Mulier, J.Rutten, C.Wittevrongel and
W.De Loecker

The oestradiol receptor concentrations increased
with age in primary breast carcinoma, while the
progesterone receptor levels remained unaffected.
Above the age of 70, all tumours examined proved
to contain oestradiol receptors. Light micros-
copical analysis was unable to relate the receptor positive tumours to any specific or predominant cellular structure. Presurgical radiotherapy with 20 G ray (Cobalt therapy source)
significantly reduced the oestradiol receptor
concentrations by 55% (n=54) while the progesterone receptor concentrations were even more affected and were reduced by 70% (n=43). Prebiop-
tic radiotherapy with 8 G ray added to a presurgical 20 G ray irradiation accentuated the reduction of the oestradiol- and progesterone receptor concentrations. The application of an additional 1 G ray resulted in a reduction of the
oestradiol- and progesterone receptors by 1.7
fmol/mg protein and 4.6 fmol/mg protein respectively. Statistical analysis of the examined
populations made by the Mann-Whitney U test
proved highly significant.

The reduction in steroid receptor concentrations
occurring after radiotherapy is important when
considering the hormone dependancy of the tumor.

Afdelingen Gezwelziekten, Gynaecologische Gezwelziekten en Biochemie, Fakulteit Geneeskunde,
Universiteit te Leuven, 3000 LOUVAIN, Belgium.

102

HYDROXY-9-METHYL-2-ELLIPTICINIUM (NSC 264-137)
IN 100 CASES OF OSSEOUS METASTASES FROM BREAST
CANCER
P. Juret, Y. Le Talaer, J.E. Couette and
T. Delozier

The authors report the analysis of 100 patients
with osseous metastases from breast cancer treated with Hydroxy-9-Methyl-2-Ellipticinium. All
these patients were previously given hormonal
treatments (castration followed by tamoxifen
when premenopausal, tamoxifen alone when post-
menopausal) and 38 of them received other chemical drugs prior to H9M2E. An objective response
was obtained in 16 of them, the longest of these
remissions reaching 18 months at the present time.
The main characteristic of this chemical drug is
its lack of hematologic toxicity, a property
which makes it useful in case of marrow insufficiency as a result either of marrow metastatic
involvement, or of the toxic effect of other
chemical agents.

Centre François Baclesse, Route de Lion-sur-mer,
14021 Caen Cedex, France.

103

THERAPY OF SMALL CELL BRONCHOGENIC CARCINOMA WITH CIS-
PLATINUM, VP 16-213 AND ADRIAMYCIN. J. Klastersky, C.
Nicaise, E. Longeval and EORTC Lung Cancer Working Party
(Belgium)

Cis-platinum (CDDP) 60 mg/m2, IV, day 1; VP 16-213, 125
mg/m2, iv, days 1, 2, 3; and adriamycin (ADM) 45 mg/m2,
IV, day 1, were used for remission induction in small cell
bronchogenic carcinoma (SCBC). Therapy was given every
three weeks and patients were evaluated after 2 courses.
22 patients with extensive diseases and 8 patients with
limited disease were studied. The median age was 58 years
and the male/female ratio was 25/7. The median performance status (Karnofsky) was 80%.

	N° evaluable patients	N° and % responses CR	PR	CR + PR
Extensive disease	19	4(22)	12(63)	16(94)
Limited disease	8	5(62)	3(37)	8(100)
Total	27	9(33)	15(55)	24(89)

The overall response rate was thus 24 out of 27 evaluable
patients; 9 (33%) complete remissions have been
observed mostly in patients with limited disease. If all
the patients in the present series (including 3 early
deaths) are considered, the response rate is 24/30 (80%).
Neutropenia (WBC<1.500) was seen in 11 patients and
severe thrombocytopenia (platelets< 20.000) was seen in
1 patient.
Renal toxicity (serum creatinine rise > 2.0 mg%) was seen
in 5 patients and was reversible in all of them. The GI
toxicity, consisting of nausea and vomiting, was seen
in most patients but was moderate in intensity.
Although it is early to evaluate the survival in this
series, it appears that the combination of CDDP, VP 16-213
and ADM is highly effective for remission induction in
SCBC.

Institut Jules Bordet, rue Héger-Bordet 1, Brussels,
Belgium

104

PHASE II TRIAL WITH N-(PHOSPHONOACETYL)-L-ASPARTATE (PALA)
IN ADVANCED MALIGNANT MELANOMA, U.R.Kleeberg, D.Kisner, P.
Rümke, J.H.Mulder, J.Revuz, E.Macher, B. Czarnetzki,
D.Thomas, and M. Rozencweig.

PALA is a synthetic antimetabolite with striking anticancer properties in experimental solid tumors. Its activity against advanced malignant melanoma was evaluated in
a cooperative phase II clinical trial. The drug was given
as a 60-min iv infusion at a daily dose of 2.5 g/m2 for 2
consecutive days.Courses were repeated every 2 weeks. The
protocol called for dose escalations by increments of 20%
if no toxicity was encountered. Patients with prior chemotherapy, creatinine levels > 1.2 mg/dl and/or CNS metastases were not eligible for entering the trial. Of 27 eligible patients, 18 were evaluable for response, 6 were too
early and 3 were not evaluable because of protocol viola-
tions (2) or early death (1). Among evaluable patients,
men and women were equally represented, median age was 56
years (range: 44-74), and median performance status on the
Karnofsky scale was 100 (range:50-100).The median number
of courses per patient amounted to 3 (range:2-8).Three patients with soft tissue lesions experienced partial remission (>50%).In 2 of these, response duration from initiation of therapy lasted 12 and 17 weeks respectively.
In the third responding patient, residual disease was surgically removed after 3 courses. All but one of the 18
evaluable patients showed minor to moderate toxic effects
consisting of cutaneous toxicity (13), stomatitis (6),
nausea and vomiting (6), diarrhea (5), vulvitis (1),proc-
titis (1), conjunctivitis (1), and somnolence (1). There
was no evidence of drug-related myelosuppression. Thus,
PALA has some efficacy against advanced malignant melanoma. Full assessment of this antitumor activity must await
further evaluation and additional patient accrual. At
this dose schedule, the drug is well tolerated. Its lack
of hematologic toxicity makes it attractive for combination chemotherapy regimens.

EORTC, Malignant Melanoma Cooperative Group.

105

PHASE II TRIAL WITH N-(PHOSPHONOACETYL)-L-ASPARTATE (PALA)
IN ADVANCED MALIGNANT MELANOMA, U.R.Kleeberg, D.Kisner, P.
Rümke, J.H.Mulder, J.Revuz, E.Macher, D.Thomas, and
M. Rozencweig.

PALA is a synthetic antimetabolite with striking anticancer properties in experimental solid tumors. Its activity against advanced malignant melanoma was evaluated in
a cooperative phase II clinical trial. The drug was given
as a 30-min iv infusion at a daily dose of 2.5 g/m2 for 2
consecutive days.Courses were repeated every 2 weeks. The
protocol called for dose escalations by increments of 20%
if no toxicity was encountered. Patients with prior chemotherapy, creatinine levels $\geq$ 1.2 mg/dl and/or CNS metastases were not eligible for entering the trial. Of 27 eligible patients, 18 were evaluable for response, 6 were too
early and 3 were not evaluable because of protocol viola-
tions (2) or early death (1). Among evaluable patients,
men and women were equally represented, median age was 56
years (range: 44-74), and median performance status on the
Karnofskyscale was 100 (range: 50-100). The median number
of courses per patient was   3 (range: 2-8). Three patients with soft tissue lesions experienced partial remission (>50%).In 2 of these, response duration from initiation of therapy lasted 12 and 17 weeks respectively.
In the third responding patient, residual disease was surgically removed after 3 courses. All but one of the 18
evaluable patients showed minor to moderate toxic effects
consisting of cutaneous toxicity (13), stomatitis (6),
nausea and vomiting (6), diarrhea (5), vulvitis (1),proc-
titis (1), conjunctivitis (1), and somnolence (1). There
was no evidence of drug-related myelosuppression. Thus,
PALA has some efficacy against advanced malignant melanoma. Full assessment of this antitumor activity must await
further evaluation and additional patient accrual. At
this dose schedule, the drug is well tolerated. Its lack
of hematologic toxicity makes it attractive for combination chemotherapy regimens.

EORTC, Malignant Melanoma Cooperative Group.

107

STUDY OF ENVIRONMENTAL FACTORS AND PRIMARY LUNG CANCER.
J.P.Kleisbauer, F.Bonnevay, A.Bettendorf, J.Colonna,
P.Laval

One hundred successive cases of primary lung cancer in
patients who had lived for at least the last ten years in
Marseilles were studied as a function of their residence
(by municipal "arrondissement") and comparison with the
degree of pollution.
Average patient age was 60 to 70 years; non-smokers represented 5% of the study group. 51% presented a history
of chronic bronchitis, and 14% had a direct ascendant who
had had cancer.
Four studies were conducted using census figures from the
I.N.S.E.E.

	1954	1962	1968	1975
Population living in polluted zone	66.3%	60.1%	58%	51%
Number of subjects with cancer living in this zone	67%	74.1%	69.9%	69%

These results show that a significant number of the pa-
tietts studied had lived in a city district in which there
was above-average pollution due to smoke and nonspecific
dust particles.

Service de Pneumo-phtisiologie, Hôpital Michel Lévy,
84a rue de Lodi, 13006 Marseille, France

106

COMBINATION OF LEVAMISOLE IMMUNOTHERAPY WITH CONVEN-
TIONAL TREATMENTS IN BREAST CANCER. Pentti Klefström,
Pentti Gröhn, Erkki Heinonen, Paul Holsti, Lauri Nuortio.

The immunocompetence of patients has been proved to
correlate positively with the treatment response to
radio- and chemotherapy. In this study Levamisole
was used in combination with conventional treatments
in breast cancer. Seventy-two stage II patients were
randomized from the start of postoperative radiotherapy to receive double-blind intermittent treatment
with either placebo (32 pts) or Levamisole 2.5 mg/kg
per day (40 pts). Similarly, 59 stage III patients
received Levamisole after operation. These patients
were randomized to receive Levamisole combined with
either chemotherapy (VAC) or radiotherapy or both.
The results were compared with those of historical
controls who received postoperative radiotherapy alone.
These studies preceded randomized double-blind study of
Levamisole immunotherapy combined with polychemotherapy
(VAC) in disseminated breast cancer (101 pts), of whom
48 received Levamisole and 53 placebo. The results
suggest that Levamisole may prolong the disease-free
and the absolute survival of patients whose immunity
is weakened by age (stage II menopaused), tumor load
(stage III, stage II-III with positive nodes) or by
treatment or disease (improvement of response to
chemotherapy in patients with advanced disease who
had negative skin test to PPD before treatment).

Radiotherapy Clinic, Helsinki University Central
Hospital, Haartmaninkatu 4, 00290 Helsinki 29,
Finland

108

ABSENCE OF SHARING IDIOTYPIC CELL SURFACE DETERMINANTS
IN A PATIENT WITH MULTIPLE MYELOMA AND SEZARY'S SYNDROME.
P.M. Kövary, I. Schedel.

Monoclonal immunoglobulinemia has repeatedly been observed in patients with Sezary's syndrome. Sharing of
idiotypic determinants of monoclonal serum immunoglobulins
and of autologous cell surface membrane immunoglobulins
of Sezary-cells might provide a relationship between both.
3 months after the detection of multiple myeloma (IgG,
kappa) Sezary's syndrome developed in a 75 year old
patient (W.B.).An antiserum directed against idiotypic
determinants of the monoclonal serum protein was prepared
after immunisation of rabbits. No reactivity was demonstrable with cell surface determinants of autologous peripheral blood lymphocytes by direct and indirect immunofluorescence technique. From the preliminary results it
may not be concluded that Sezary' syndrome and multiple
myeloma in our patient are related.

P.D. Dr. med. P.M. Kövary
Universitäts-Hautklinik
D-44 Münster
West-Germany

109

RESTORATION AND STIMULATION OF DELAYED CUTANEOUS HYPERSEN-
SITIVITY IN CANCER PATIENTS AFTER A SHORT-COURSE TREATMENT
WITH C 1740. J.M.Lang, C.Giron, F.Oberling

C 1740 is a glycoprotein extract from klebsiella pneumo-
niae (Laboratoires Cassenne, Centre de Recherche Roussel
UCLAF). It was given orally at a dose of 8 mg/day for 15
days (10 patients) or 7 days (8 patients) to 18 selected
patients of both sexes, ranging in age from 16 to 68 years.
Patients were either untreated and evaluated at the time
of diagnosis (4 with Hodgkin's disease, 4 with non-Hodgkin
lymphomas, 5 with solid tumors), or relapsing at distance
of previous treatment (2 patients), or patients with Hodgkin's disease in unmaintained complete remission (3 patients). These patients were unlikely to show spontaneous
recovery or increase of skin reactivity during the trial,
and they were given no other drug. Delayed cutaneous hypersensitivity (DCH) was tested just before and after immunostimulation using a standardized and reproducible de-
vice which allows the simultaneous injection of 7 recall
antigens (Multitest, Institut Mérieux). Skin reactions
were evaluated after 48 hours by measuring two crossed diameters of the induration. DCH was clearly restored in 9/11
anergic or hypoergic patients, and clearly enhanced in
6/7 patients with positive reactions. Immuno-restoration
or stimulation was assayed in each patient by the number
of positive skin reactions to the 7 antigens and by the
calculative score defined by the sum of the two diameters
of induration for all positive reactions. This study not
only demonstrates the immuno-restoring and stimulating
properties of C 1740 but also shows that the mechanism(s)
of skin anergy in cancer patients including HD may be
overcome by a short course of immunotherapy.

Clinique des Maladies du Sang, Hôpital de Hautepierre,
67098 Strasbourg, France.

110

SURGICAL TREATMENT OF PULMONARY METASTASES IN ADULT
PATIENTS AT THE GUSTAVE ROUSSY INSTITUTE. T. Le Chevalier,
J. Rouesse, G. Lemoine, R. Arriagada

From 1972 to 1979, 86 thoracotomies were performed for
metastases in 75 adult patients (48 with carcinoma, 27
with sarcoma). The population was composed of 42 men and
33 women aged 15 to 72 years.
Six patients underwent bilateral thoracotomy (simultaneous for one, and at a three-week interval for the other
five). Three patients had two iterative thoracotomies
and one patient three thoracotomies.
Operative mortality was 1.1% (1/86); four benign lesions
were found.
Three patients had a pneumonectomy, 24 a lobectomy, 5 a
segmentectomy, 1 a pleurectomy, 5 a mediastinal adenec-
tomy and 40 wedge resections.
Fifteen patients has an explorative thoracotomy with or
without limited resection.
Nineteen patients presented a pulmonary recurrence 3 to
24 months after the thoracotomy, but 32 patients are
alive and free of disease from 2 to 132 months following
thoracotomy (mean 23 months).
We discuss the indications for surgical pulmonary meta-
stasectomy in solid tumors of adult patients as part of
the general strategy for metastatic cancer treatment.

Institut Gustave Roussy
Hautes Bruyères, rue Camille Desmoulins
94800 Villejuif, France

111

RADIOLOGIC ASPECTS OF NON-HODGKIN'S LYMPHOMAS OF THE DI-
GESTIVE TRACT. P.Lecomte, J.N.Bruneton, G.Lesbats, J.Eliot,
J.Bourry, M.Schneider

Based on 47 personal observations and the review of 1200
cases reported in the literature, the authors discuss the
radiologic aspects of these infrequent localisations,
which generally present certain specific characteristics:
image size greater than or equal to 10 cm in over two-
thirds of cases; a general lack of correlation between the
limited extent of the clinical signs and the considerable
degree of radiologic findings; the exceptional character
of stenotic forms; the frequency of combined forms (one
third of all cases).
Lymphomas of the stomach are the most frequent and occur
in various forms : ulcerations (52%), defects (24.3%),
rigidity without stenosis (26.2%), hyperrugosity (17.6%).
Small bowel involvement is more rare, and also occurs in
several forms : infiltrating (54%), ulcerating (36.1%),
mesenteric (29.6%), multinodular (22.7%) and endo- and
exoluminal (2%).
Lymphomas of the colon and rectum are rare, the major
forms being : nodular (43.2%), infiltrating (23.7%), lacu-
nar (defects) (21.6%) and endo- and exoluminal (15.5%).
Esophageal lymphoma is exceptional, occurring in nodular
forms which are generally the result of propagation from
a gastric lesion.

Centre Antoine-Lacassagne, 36 Voie Romaine, 06054 Nice
Cedex, France

112

LEVAMISOLE IN THE MAINTENANCE THERAPY OF ACUTE
MYELOID LEUKAEMIA Marja Lehtinen* for the
Finnish Leukaemia Group

Finnish Leukaemia Group (FLG) has carried out
a randomized multicentre trial to study the
effect of Levamisole on the remission maintained
with daily 6-mercaptopurine and weekly
methotrexate.The trial was started in Dec.73
and closed in Aug.76.In remission,25 adult AML
patients were randomized to receive only chemotherapy,26 patients to receive also Levamisole.
Levamisole was given on three consecutive days
fortnightly.The groups were similar with regard
to the age of the patients,to the type of the
leukaemia and to the amount of cytostatic agents
given during induction.Analysis of the remission
curves by the summary χ^2- test revealed that
patients receiving Levamisole have significantly better remission duration than patients
treated with chemotherapy only (p=0.033).There
are four long-term survivors in the Levamisole
group with remissions lasting from four to six
years.
*Tampere Central Hospital,33520 Tampere 52,Fin
land
Members of the Finnish Leukaemia Group:M.Lehti-
nen,P.Ahrenberg,A.Hänninen,E.Ikkala,R.Lahtinen,
A.Levanto,I.Palva,A.Rajamäki,S.Rosengård,T.Ruu-
tu,S.Sarna,O.Selroos,T.Timonen,E.Waris,C.Wasa-
stjerna,J.Vilpo,P.Vuopio.
Univ.Hospitals of Tampere,Helsinki,Kuopio,Tur-
ku and Oulu,Central Hospitals in Joensuu,Kok-
kola,Lappeenranta and Vaasa,Dept.of Public
Health Sciences,Univ.of Helsinki

113

SECRETION OF THYMIDINE (TdR) BY NORMAL AND ACTIVATED PERITONEAL MACROPHAGES. F.J. Lejeune, R. Arnould, A. Vercammen-Grandjean, A. Libert.

Previous work from our laboratory demonstrated 1) the presence of macrophages (MØ) in human and mouse malignant melanomas, 2) the secretion of soluble factors inhibiting tritiated thymidine uptake by melanoma cells in vitro. Present work further shows that normal and activated MØ secrete TdR in vitro. BDF_1, GIF, Balb/c and C57bl mouse MØ showed a lack of TdR Kinase (TK) activity, and their culture media exerted a significant inhibition of H_3TdR uptake by melanoma cells. Cultured B16 melanoma cells, L cells and SV40 transformed MØ (IC21, J774A, P388D1) exhibited the reverse : high TK activity and absence of H_3TdR inhibition in melanoma cells by their supernatants. Since MØ lack   TK, they should produce unincorporated TdR. Thin layer chromatography demonstrated the presence of TdR in the 72 H culture media from normal MØ and from glucan activated MØ. No TdR was detected in transformed MØ spent culture media. That TdR secretion results from an active metabolic process was demonstrated : 1) incorporation of H_3 Orotic acid by normal MØ was followed by the secretion of H_3TdR in the culture medium, 2) H_3TdR monophosphate was dephosphorylated into H_3TdR by MØ and released. Since 10^{-3} mg/ml TdR can be secreted in 72 Hrs by 10^6 MØ/ml, this phenomenon not only produces   competition with H_3TdR, but also can inhibit DNA synthesis in tumour cells and lymphocytes merely through the mecanism of TdR blockade.

Laboratory of Oncology and Experimental Surgery, Institut Jules Bordet, Université Libre de Bruxelles. 1000 Bruxelles. Belgium.

114

MALIGNANT LYMPHOMA OF SMALL CLEAVED CELLS. A RETROSPECTIVE ANALYSIS. P. Lenner, E. Lundgren, L. Damber.

In a retrospective series of 302 patients with non-Hodgkin's lymphoma, admitted between 1959 and 1975, 84 (28%) had tumours with small cleaved cell morphology. 47 of these (55%) were nodular. 48 patients (57%) presented in clinical stage III-IV (majority were not staged by lymphography, none by laparotomy). 17 patients (21%) had systemic symptoms. 35% of patients had bone marrow involvement assessed by aspiration biopsy with cytologic and histologic examination. 15% disclosed peripheral blood involvement at admission and an additional 14% developed this sign during the course of the disease. 92% of patients in stage I or II achieved complete remission after therapy (mostly radiotherapy). The majority (70%) relapsed, with a median time to first relapse of 21 months. First relapse often (61%) appeared in distant sites in relation to the primary tumour. Median survival in all stages was 34 months. Patients with nodular lesions survived significantly longer (median 52 months) than those with diffuse tumours (median 15 months).

It is concluded that lymphoma of small cleaved cells is very often (always?) a systemic disease with high propensity for dissemination, often of leukemic type. Albeit often very sensitive to treatment this tumour has a strong tendency to relapse, and virtually all patients succumb to the disease sooner or later. Survival is, however, relatively favorable as compared the more aggressive, large cell lymphomas.

Department of Oncology, University of Umeå, S-901 87 Umeå, Sweden.

115

COMPARATIVE STUDIES OF TWO ANTITUMOR ANTHRACYCLINES : INTER ACTION OF ADRIAMYCIN (ADR) AND AD-32 WITH DNA. M.Levin, M.Israel, M.Potmesil , R.Silber (Introduced by F.Muggia)

N-trifluoroacetyl ADR-14 valerate (AD-32), an anolog of ADR, and ADR have been studied with respect to their interaction with DNA, using the alkaline elution method of Kohn and co-workers (BBA 562 : 32-40,1979). This technique permits the identification of single-stranded DNA breaks, DNA-DNA, or DNA-protein crosslinks, and is based on the elution rate of isotope-labeled DNA through polyvinyl-chloride filters at pH 12.1. In experiments summarized in a previous abstract (Levin et al; Blood 54:224a,1979) L1210 mouse leukemia cells were exposed at equitoxic doses of AD-32 (13.8µM) and ADR (2.8µM) for one hour. Both agents caused a high frequency of protein-associated DNA breaks (0.684 and 1.035 per 10^6 nucleotides, respectively) and a lesser number of DNA-DNA and DNA-protein cross links. Similarly, in vivo experiments using the ascitic form of DBA/3 mouse lymphoma demonstrated all three types of interaction 1 hour after a single IV injection of either agent.
These results document DNA damage occurring in sensitive cell lines following AD-32 which are qualitatively similar to those induced by ADR. Further information may be obtained through studies of resistant cell lines, and also by investigating the kinetics of repair following damage. The alkaline elution method appears to be a useful technique to explore differences between close analogs within the same family of compounds.

New York University Medical Center, Division of Oncology, 550 First Avenue, New York, N.Y. 10016, USA

Corrected version of abstract number 141 of the December 1979 meeting of the Society of Medical Oncology.

116

THE EFFECT OF ADRIAMYCIN, AD32, AND THEIR METABOLITES ON THE DNA OF L1210 CELLS IN VITRO. M. Levin, R. Silber, M. Israel and M. Potmesil (Introduced by F. Muggia).
N-trifluoroacetyladriamycin-14-valerate (AD32), an analogue of the anthracycline adriamycin (ADR), has greater anti-tumor activity than ADR against a spectrum of experimental tumors and is now in clinical trials. ADR and its major metabolite adriamycinol (AMNOL) bind and intercalate with DNA. In contrast, AD32 and its metabolites N-trifluoroacetyl adriamycin (AD41) and N-trifluoroacetyl adriamycinol (AD92) bind minimally, if at all, to DNA. Exponentially growing L1210 leukemia cells were labeled with ^{3}H-thymidine (0.1 µCi/ml). These cells were then exposed to drugs for 1 hour at 37°C at a concentration of 9 x 10^5 cells/ml. The following drugs were used at equitoxic µM concentrations: AD32 (13.8), AD41 (9.0), AD92 (43.7), ADR (2.8), and AMNOL (26.9). Drug-treated as well as control cells were examined by the DNA alkaline elution method. The results indicate that these drugs caused a high frequency of protein associated DNA breaks and DNA protein crosslinks. Despite the absence of the direct interaction of AD32 and its metabolites with DNA. these drugs produced DNA alteration comparable to those ascribed to intercalating anthracyclines. Cell extracts were examined with HPLC and no evidence of conversion of AD32 to ADR or AMNOL was found in L1210 cells. AD41 produced the greatest number of DNA protein associated breaks/10^6 nucleotides (3.97) followed by AD92 (2.00), ADR (0.97), AD32 (0.93), and AMNOL (0.60). These findings reflect the greater cytotoxicity observed with AD41. The similar effects on DNA macromolecules observed with intercalating and non-DNA binding anthracyclines are consistent with the concept that mechanisms other than direct interaction with DNA play a role in the toxic effects of these compounds.

Department of Medicine, New York University Medical Center, 550 First Avenue, New York, NY   10016.

117

MONITORING REMISSION IN ACUTE LYMPHOBLASTIC LEUKAEMIA (ALL) IN ADULTS. T.A. Lister and P. Elliott

Relapse of ALL has occurred in 32 of 44 adults achieving complete remission (CR) at St. Bartholomew's Hospital between January 1973 and March 1978. Patients were followed up with fortnightly clinical and peripheral blood examination and bi-monthly bone marrow (BM) and cerebrospinal fluid (CSF) examinations. This report is based on data from 33 initial relapses in 30 patients. Two have been excluded because of insufficient data.
Relapse was detected in the BM alone in 16 cases, in the central nervous system (CNS) alone in 6, in the testis in 4 and in the skin in 1. Simultaneous relapse occurred in the BM and CNS twice and in the BM and testis once. It was suspected on clinical grounds in 24 out of 33 occasions and in 5 of these was suspected a fortnight previously. Fifteen out of 19 BM relapses were symptomatic. All were anticipated from peripheral blood abnormalities. BM aspiration had been normal in 11 out of 12 cases within 8 weeks and suspicious in only one (8%). It was normal in the remaining of them within the preceding 12 weeks. Six CNS relapses were symptomatic and 2 were detected on CSF examination. Routine CSF examination had been normal in 5 within 8 weeks but not performed in 3. All testicular relapses were detected clinically and only one was symptomatic. The skin relapse was detected clinically and confirmed histologically.
Regular clinical and peripheral blood examination remains the best means of detecting relapse in ALL in adults. BM and CSF examination should be performed only when special grounds for suspicion exist.

Dr. T.A. Lister, Imperial Cancer Research Fund, Dept. of Medical Oncology, St. Bartholomew's Hospital, London EC1A 7BE, England

118

TERMINAL HALF-LIFE MODIFICATIONS IN PATIENTS RECEIVING REPEATED HIGH DOSE METHOTREXATE. F.Lokiec, C.Gisselbrecht, M.Marty, Y.Najean, M.Boiron

Unexpected toxicity unrelated to alterations in renal function tests in patients receiving high dose methotrexate (HDMTX) by repeated courses prompted a prospective study of pharmacokinetics in those patients.
MTX plasma levels were monitored using a radioimmunoassay in 13 patients treated by repeated courses of MTX. In no case was the dose escalated during the therapy. In all cases, MTX was administered by push IV (1/3 dose) followed by a 4 hour infusion (2/3 of the dose) in patients with alkaline diuresis. Rescue with CF was used in every case. As previously described, a ten-fold variation in the peak plasma levels could be observed. Furthermore, a progressive increase in terminal half-life was observed in 11/13 patients (84%). Although this increase was of limited extent in most patients (7-10%/course), it reached 120% in one patient with normal renal function tests.
Such results demonstrate induction of subclinical cumulative alterations in renal function by MTX and/or HDMTX. Such damage implies that :
1) detailed pharmacokinetics (8 dosages) are warranted every 3 courses in patients receiving HDMTX.
2) Escalation of doses can lead to unexpected toxicity without constant therapeutic improvement.
3) Pharmacological simulation has to take such modifications of MTX clearance into account in order to predict modifications of administered doses along repeated courses.

Institut de Recherches sur les Leucémies, Hôpital Saint-Louis, 2 Place du Dr.Fournier, 75010 Paris, France

119

CISPLATIN-VP16 COMBINATION IN NON SMALL CELL (NSC) BRONCHOGENIC CARCINOMA. E.Longeval, P.Balasse, D.Becquart, J.L.Bernheim, A.Boute, R.Daubies, P.Dierckx, P.Libert, M.Mairesse, J.Michel, C.Nicaise, R.Paridaens, J.Thiriaux, A.Verhest, D.Weerts, Y.Kenis, J.Klastersky,EORTC Lung Cancer Working Party

Ninety-seven patients with NSC bronchogenic carcinoma were treated from February 1979 with a combination of cisplatin (60 mg/m^2, day 1) and VP16(120 mg/m^2, day 3, 5, 7, given by i.v. infusion). This schedule was repeated q 3-4 weeks and evaluation was made at 6-7 weeks. Final results will be presented and discussed. So far, 60 patients have been adequately evaluated. Median age was 61 years and median performance status (Karnofsky) was 70. Only 6 patients had received prior chemotherapy. The total response rate was 38%, with 4 CR and 19 PR. Patients with loco-regional disease responded much better than those with disseminated disease (52 vs 28%). One CR was obtained in the case of a patient with bilateral lung metastases. Response rate was nearly similar in squamous cell (36%) and adenocarcinoma (44%). Nausea, vomiting, and alopecia were almost universal. Mild and transient renal failure developed in 2 cases. Significant thrombopenia (<50,000 /mm3) was observed in 2 other cases. Leucopenia, however, was the major hematologic toxicity. Median WBC nadir after the first course was 2,500 /mm3, and a WBC count under 1000/mm3 was noted in 20% of the patients. One of them developed fatal sepsis. The length of the 4 CR is respectively 14, 12$^+$, 10$^+$, and 5$^+$ months. Definite statements concerning survival cannot yet be established.

Institut Jules Bordet, Rue Héger-Bordet,1, 1000 Brussels, Belgium

120

A NEW HIGHLY WATER SOLUBLE PLATINUM ANTITUMOR COMPOUND (PHIC) WITH LOWER TOXICITY AND HIGHER THERAPEUTIC INDEX THAN CISPLATIN. J.P. Macquet

A new platinum antitumor compound abbreviated PHIC (Platinum 1,2-diaminocycloHexane IsoCitrate) was synthetized from the diaquo species of 1,2-diaminocyclohexane Pt(II), Pt(DAC) and the isocitrate ion. The analytical results indicate a 1:1 (ligand : Pt) complex. The water solubility of PHIC is greater than 1500 mg/ml.
Toxicity of PHIC (LDo = 250 μm/kg) is much lower than that of cisplatin (LDo = 30 μm/kg) in mice. PHIC did not induce any nephrotoxicity in mice as revealed by histopathologic evaluation of the kidneys at a dose of 150 mg/kg, whereas kidney tubular necrosis is detected for cisplatin at a dose of 8 mg/kg.
Antitumoral properties at the maximum tolerated dose in experimental ascites tumors, leukaemia L1210 (10^5 cells, treatment on day 1) and sarcoma S180 (10^6 cells, treatment on day 1), are greater for PHIC (L1210 : ILS = 232 %, 30 % cures ; S180 : ILS = 126 %, 40 % cures) at a dose of 125 mg/kg than for cisplatin (L1210 : ILS = 100 %, no cure ; S180 : ILS = 65 %, no cure) at a dose of 8 mg/kg. Therapeutic indexes (TI = LD50/ID90) on these two tumors are significantly higher for PHIC compared with cisplatin.

COMPARISON BETWEEN PHIC AND CISPLATIN

	PHIC	CISPLATIN
Hydrosolubility	> 1500 mg/ml	2 mg/ml
Antitumor properties		
a. therapeutic index		
- L1210	25	6.5
- S180	17.5	6
b. cures	yes	no
Nephrotoxicity (mice)	no	yes

Laboratoire de Pharmacologie et de Toxicologie Fondamentales du C.N.R.S., 205, route de Narbonne, 31078 TOULOUSE CEDEX, France.

121

NON SPECIFIC INTERACTIONS IN COMPETITIVE CEA RADIO-IMMUNOASSAY
* R. Maiolini, ** J.P. Cassuto, *** B.P. Krebs and * R. Masseyeff

A preliminary correlation study of carcinoembryonic antigen (CEA) levels obtained by radio-immunoassay (RIA, direct competitive assay) and enzyme-immunoassay (EIA, non competitive sandwich assay after extraction) showed a good correlation (r = 0.94, number of cases 144). However, three kinds of discrepancies were observed : 1) a systematic difference in the ratio of obtained values which are roughly threefold greater in the RIA assay than in the EIA one ; 2) differences observed in the lower range, especially when the CEA levels measured by the EIA were inferior to 20 µg/l ; 3) strongly discrepant results in a limited number of sera. Further samples were assayed by both techniques. Two highly discrepant sera (2.7 and 1.3 µg/l by the EIA/CEA and 72 and 130 µg/l by the RIA respectively) were extensively studied. 1) The RIA assay of dilutions of these sera showed no parallelism with the standard curve ; 2) Preliminary extraction of these sera by acid buffer at 70ºC followed by the RIA led to normal values ; 3) Addition of pooled rabbit normal serum or rabbit IgG also led to normal values. From these data, these discrepancies were interpreted as resulting from the interference of antiglobulin factors. The assay of 81 sera containing rheumatoid factors showed interference in 9 sera. It was concluded from this result and from neutralisation studies that the main factor involved is the occurrence of anti-rabbit gammaglobulin.
Thus, occurrence of antiglobulinic factors directed against the animal species providing the antiserum represents a neglected drawback in all competitive RIA or EIA.

* INSERM FRA 12, Laboratoire d'Immunologie du CHU, 06034 Nice Cédex
** Clinique Médicale du CHU (Pr. P. Audoly), 06031 Nice Cédex
*** Centre Antoine Lacassagne, 06054 Nice Cédex

122

THE MERITS OF THE ILIAC CREST BIOPSY IN STAGING OF HUMAN MALIGNANCY. Ch. Manegold, D. Fritze, R. Herrmann, B. Krempien

The purpose of our ongoing study was to evaluate the merits of the iliac crest biopsy in tumor staging of various human neoplasms.Approximately 150 biopsies were examind including cases of metastatic breast cancer (34), Non-Hodgkin-Lymphoma (36), Hodgkin-Lymphoma (15), plasmocytoma (11), primary bone tumors (9), colon carcinoma (5), acute (6) and chronic leucemia (10),and cases with suspicion of hematologic disorder(24). The biopsies were obtained unilateraly utiliz - ing the biopsy technique devised by Jamshidi and Swain. For light microscopy undecalcified bone sections were used which had been stained as outlined by Masson/Goldner.Results: Neoplastic bone involvement was found in 49 % of metastatic breast carcinoma, in 20 % of Hodgkin-Lymphoma, and in 47 % of Non-Hodgkin-Lymphoma. By consider ing the bone marrow cellularity, the amount of connective tissue and the secondary changes in bone tissue of the specimen, a diagnosis in a suspected hematologic disorder could be con - firmed in almost 50 % of the biopsies. Conclu - sions: The Jamshidi iliac crest biopsy technique which is simple to perform and can be done on an in - and outpatient basis seems to be a very useful method in diagnosis and staging in Hod- gkin-Lymphoma, Non-Hodgkin-Lymphoma and various primary hematologic disorders as well as in ad- vanced solid neoplasia such as carcinoma of the breast. Updated results will be presented.

Dr. med. Ch. Manegold, Medizinische Universitäts klinik und Tumorzentrum Heidelberg, Bergheimer Str. , D- 6900 Heidelberg, West Germany.

123

CONTINUOUS 5-DAY INFUSION VINDESINE (VDS) IN THE TREATMENT OF ADVANCED LEUKEMIAS AND HEMATOSARCOMAS. D. Maraninchi, J.A. Gastaut, N. Tubiana and Y. Carcassonne

-VDS in IV push has been shown as an effective agent in the treatment of Leukemias and Hematosarcomas (1). The short plasma half-life of VDS (2) suggests that continuous infusion can improve the therapeutic results by maintaining a constant plasma level.
-Treatment schedule associated one IV bolus (2mg/m2) for a pharmacokinetic study, followed by a 5-day infusion. The infusion was done in a central catheter, with a peristaltic pump and repeated every ten days. 38 infusions have been given at doses between 0.7 and 1 mg/m2/day.
-21 patients (pts) entered this study ; all had advanced and measurable disease, resistant to usual chemotherapies, including other vinca alkaloïd agents. 11 pts had Leukemia and 10 had Hematosarcomas.
-18 pts are evaluable for response : Partial Responses (PR) (50% Tumor regression ≥1 month) were seen in 6 (33%) -4/11 Leukemia and 2/7 Hematosarcomas. Minor regression (25% Tumor regression or less than 1 month) was observed in 7 pts (39%). Progressive disease was seen in 5 pts (28%). Instead frequent responses (72%) they were usually brief, and only one pt is in continuous remission after 5 months. Myelosuppression included thrombocytopenia in 6 pts and Leukopenia in 5 pts. Other side effects were alopecia in 5 pts (25%), mild neurotoxocity in 5 pts, digestive symptomes in 4 pts. Phlebitis was observed in the 2 pts for whom treatment had been initiated in a peripheral vein.
-Our results suggest that VDS given in this manner 1) is not associated with severe toxicity 2) is effective in the treatment of advanced Leukemias and Hematosarcomas. 3) More prolonged responses might be obtained by combination chemotherapy including VDS infusion.

(1) Cancer Chemother. Pharmacol. 2, 247 - 255 (1979)
(2) Cancer Research 37, 2603 - 2607 (1977)

INSTITUT PAOLI-CALMETTES - Clinique des Maladies du Sang. Marseille - FRANCE.

124

99m Tc BONE SCINTIGRAPHY IN CHRONIC MYELOPROLIFERATIVE DISORDERS AND ACUTE LEUKEMIAS. D. Maraninchi , J. Pasquier, N. Tubiana, R. Sauvan, J.A. Gastaut and Y. Carcassonne

Bone scintigraphy (99m Tc M.D.P.) has been performed in 43 adult patients with blood diseases. 26 were male and 17 were female ; mean age was 55 Yr (range from 18 to 76). 28 patients had chronic myeloproliferative syndromes : 20 had chronic granulocytic leukemia (CGL) of whom 15 were in blastic crisis (B.C.) ; 4 had primary myelofibrosis, 3 had primary thrombocythemia and 1 had polycythemia vera. 15 patients had acute blood diseases : 8 ALL, 5 ANLL, 1 leukemic malignant lymphoma and 1 pre-leukemic myelofibrosis.
In 20 CGL all patients in B.C. had abnormal Tc scan with intensive hyperfixation. Patients in chronic phase had normal Tc scan, except one. In other chronic myeloproliferative syndromes Tc scans were only positive in 4 patients with primary myelofibrosis.
In acute leukemias patients in complete remission had normal Tc scan. Hyperfixation was observed in most of the patients in blastic phase. Abnormal Tc scan was strongly related with the presence of fibrosis in the bone marrow biopsy : 19 patients with myelofibrosis had hyperfixation. 16 out of these 19 patients had blastic involvement.
Abnormal Tc scan may reflect, as in solid tumors, the structural modification of bone secondary to the involvement by malignant cells. This involvement is often associated with fibrosis. Sequential Tc scan may represent an important method of follow-up in myeloproliferative disorders with the aim of early detection of accelerated phases.

INSTITUT PAOLI - CALMETTES, Services d'Hématologie et de Médecine Nucléaire - 232, Bd de Sainte Marguerite - 13009 MARSEILLE.

32

125

MACROMOLECULAR BINDING OF DEXAMETHASONE IN HUMAN BREAST CANCER : EVIDENCE FOR THE PRESENCE OF MINERALOCORTICOID RECEPTOR. P.M.Martin, P.H.Rolland

Corticoid (C), estrogen (E) and progestin (P) binding sites were assayed in cytosol from 356 human breast tumors. Corticoid binding measured after incubation for at least 1hr at 20° and overnight at 0° was recovered in 70 to 80% of the tumors. The effect of storage on CR, ER and PR was minimal provided tumor samples were stored in liquid nitrogen. The presence of 1 mM sodium molybdate inhibited the time-dependent decrease that occurred spontaneously in CR sites. In a study with dextran-coated charcoal adsorption technique on 236 tumors attempts were made to distinguish between glucocorticoid (GR) and mineralocorticoid (MR) binding by measuring binding sites with (a) ^{3}H-DXM displaced with cold DXM (defining CR and MR) and (b) ^{3}H-DXM displaced with a 500-fold excess of a highly specific glucocorticoid RU 26988 (defining GR only). Method (a) showed that 75% of the tumors contained CR (less than 150 fmoles/mg protein, mean = 38 fmoles/mg prot.) and that their presence was correlated (p less than 0.001) with ER and PR presence. Method (a) indicated that 1) only 32% of tumors contained CR when the specific glucocorticoid was present in excess, and 2) in 8% of the tumors, RU 26988 was unable to displace ^{3}H-DXM binding while cold aldosterone was effective. In these 8% of tumors, DXM-binding entity had the properties of a mineralocorticoid receptor : a Kd at 0° for aldosterone of 0.81 nM, a number of binding sites of 51 fmoles/mg protein low and heavy sedimentation forms in sucrose gradient analysis and a steroid specificity restricted to mineralocorticoids. These results indicate that MR is contained in a significant proportion of human breast tumors. From these, a major question remains to be answered: is hormone-dependence a complex endocrine regulation involving estrogen as well as influences from other hormones acting through their own receptors?

Laboratoire des Récepteurs Hormonaux. Faculté de Médecine de Marseille(secteur Nord), 13326 Marseille Cedex 3,France

126

A PHASE I STUDY OF BD40, ADIPYRIDOINDOLE DERIVATIVE. M.Marty, C.Jasmin, P.Pouillart, C.Gisselbrecht, E.Gouveia, E.Garcia-Giralt, H.Magdelenat, G.Mathé

Diethylaminopropyl-amino dipyridoindole (BD40) is an intercalating agent structurally related to ellipticins. A potent antitumor activity has been shown in experimental tumors (L1210, B16, Lewis, TG180, murine sarcoma and leukemia) with an interesting therapeutic index. Of interest is the lack of bone marrow depression in animals. These data prompted a phase I study in humans.
BD40 as a maleate salt was administered to pts with advanced malignancies as a 45 min infusion every two weeks. Starting dose was 0.5 mg/kg. 3 patients had to be treated at each dose level; if no grade 4-5 toxicity was observed, dosage was escalated in the following pts. Follow-up, included clinical survey as well as bone marrow, lung, cardiac, liver, renal, neurological function studies.
Doses were escalated to 25 mg/kg. Main toxicity appears to be circulatory : a 1 point drop in blood pressure was observed in 2 pts at the 13 mg/kg level. Such circulatory abnormalities were observed infrequently at the following doses. However, at the 25 mg/kg level, 2 grade 4 or 5 shocks occurred. Maximum tolerated dose as a single injection is 25 mg/kg. In no pt were GI symptoms or alopecia observed. Bone marrow depression, although of limited significance in these pts with extensive prior chemotherapy, was observed in 15% of pts. A slight increase in transaminases was observed in 1 pt at 6 mg/kg and in 2 pts at 15 mg/kg.
Responses were observed in multiple myeloma (2 pts), breast cancer (2 pts), glioblastoma (1 pt), AML (3 pts), corpus uteri (1 pt) and colorectal (3 pts).
BD40 appears to be a well tolerated anticancer agent with demonstrable activity in heavily pretreated pts. Other schedules are now under study.

° Hôp.Saint-Louis,Paris; °° Hôp.Paul-Brousse, Villejuif; °°° Institut Curie, Paris, France.

127

REH CELL LINE AS A TOOL FOR IMMUNOTHERAPY AND CHARACTERIZATION OF cALL
M.C. Martyré, M. Barel, C. Charriaut, R. Frade and C. Rosenfeld

Twenty-five patients with acute lymphoid leukemia (ALL) in remission were treated with BCG plus irradiated REH cells. Their sera were tested sequentially in a microcytotoxicity assay for the presence of antibodies against REH cells. Seventeen patients have demonstrated such antibodies. A 28 month follow-up of the patients indicated that the titer of antibodies varies from patient to patient, and for the same patient during the period of immunization. The results obtained after adequate absorptions on a pool of normal lymphocytes suggest that the immunization with REH cells raises in some ALL patients the titer of antibodies against an antigenic structure closely related to the cALL antigen. This cALL antigen has been isolated and purified from REH cells. We will report data obtained with our rabbit antiserum compared to other antisera.

This work was supported by grants from CNAMTS, DGRST (80.7.226) and UER Kremlin-Bicêtre(782)

Département de Culture et de Production de Cellules Humaines, I.C.I.G., I.N.S.E.R.M. U.50, 14 avenue Paul Vaillant Couturier, 94800 Villejuif, France

128

A RETROSPECTIVELY CONTROLLED TRIAL OF BCG ± D.T.I.C. ADJUVANT THERAPY IN LOCALLY RECURRENT MALIGNANT MELANOMA. Peter B. McCulloch and Peter B.Dent.

Eighty-seven sequentially treated patients with locally recurrent malignant melanoma (including regional nodes) were rendered surgically disease free. Group I (N=29) no adjuvant therapy, minimum follow-up 10 yrs. Group II (N=29) Connaught Laboratories BCG, 5 mgms. by Tine, rotating to all four limbs q 1 month x 2 yrs and at decreasing intervals until 5 years after initial surgery, minimum follow-up 5 years, Group III (N=29) BCG by Tine as in Group II + D.T.I.C. 850 mgm/M² I.V. at the start of immunotherapy and one further dose 28 days later, minimum follow-up 2.5 years. Adjuvant therapy was started within 12 weeks of surgery. Median survival Group I=16 mos., Group II=26 mos., Group III=21 mos. Five year true survivalGroup I, 24%, Group II, 48%. Survival curves between Group I and Group II are significantly different (p>0.05). However, the addition of D.T.I.C. to immunotherapy has decreased median survival and produces an actuarial survival curve midway between Group I and Group II. BCG immunotherapy alone appears to improve median and 5 year survival, but the addition of D.T.I.C. adds no benefit and potentially decreases the improved survival conferred by BCG alone.

McMaster University and the Ontario Cancer Foundation, Hamilton, Canada.

129

A STRATIFIED, RANDOMIZED TRIAL OF 5 F.U., ADRIAMYCIN AND CYCLOPHOSPHAMIDE ALONE OR WITH BCG IN STAGE IV BREAST CANCER. P. B.McCulloch, M.Poon, P.B. Dent and Penny Dawson.

Forty-nine women who have failed hormonal therapy and not received prior palliative chemotherapy have been divided into 6 strata for site and extent of disease. All received 500 mgm. 5 F.U./M^2, 50 mgm. Adriamycin/M^2 and 500 mgm. Cyclophosphamide/M^2 (FAC) q28 days I.V. Half were randomized to receive 5 mgm. Connaught Laboratories BCG vaccine I.D. q1 wk. x 2 mos. then q 1 month on day 21 after the chemotherapy. Numbers in each stratum are nearly equal. Minimum follow-up is 32 months. FAC alone (N=25) gave 44% stabilization (S), 12% partial response (PR) and 0% complete response (CR); median duration 7.5 mos. (4 to 22 mos.), median survival 10 mos. (3 to 31+ mos.). FAC+BCG (N=24) gave 29% S, 29% PR and 8% CR; median duration 10 mos. (4 to 26 mos.), median survival 16 mos.(3 to 38 mos.). FAC+ BCG gives borderline statistical benefit (p=0.05). The benefit appears to be conferred on those women (14/24) with plasma CEA> 5 ng/ml before starting chemotherapy + BCG (median survival 24 mos.) The other 3 subsets (FAC alone + elevated CEA, FAC+BCG with normal CEA) 29/49 cases have a median survival of 9 mos. The difference between these two survival curves shows high significance (p<0.01).

McMaster University and the Ontario Cancer Foundation, Hamilton, Canada.

130

COMBINATION CHEMOTHERAPY OF ADVANCED OVARIAN CARCINOMA WITH HEXAMETHYLMELAMINE, CYCLOPHOSPHAMIDE, METHOTREXATE AND FLUOROURACIL (HEXACAF). C. Mendiola, R. Quiben, V. Hernandez, A. Ramos, H. Cortés Funes

Fifteen consecutive patients without prior chemotherapy with advanced ovarian carcinoma were treated with a combination of hexamethylmelamine and cyclophosphamide (150 mg/m2 p.o. on days 1 to 14) + Methotrexate (40 mg/m2 IV) + Fluorouracil (600 mg/m2 IV), the last two drugs both IV on days 1 and 8; this course was repeated every 3-4 months.
The overall response rate of 13 evaluable patients with measurable disease was 53.3% (2 CR and 5 PR). Median duration for responders was 18 months for CRs and 9 months for PRs. Second look surgery was performed in two PR patients and complete removal of residual masses was performed in one of them.
Toxicity was mild, with nausea and vomiting in 80% and WBC below 2000 in 20% of patients. There were no treatment related deaths. Neurologic toxicity due to HMM was not clinically evident. Five patients resistant to this regimen were treated with a combination of Cisplatin (60 mg/m2 IV) and Adriamycin (45 mg/m2 IV). There were no objective responses.
It is concluded that the Hexa-CAF combination is an active regimen for advanced ovarian carcinoma, but the lower CR rate obtained and the further resistance to new drugs such as cisplatin and ADM must be considered in order to include these last two drugs in future first line chemotherapy regimens.

Seccion de Oncologia Médica
Hospital "1º de Octubre"
Madrid, Spain

131

TREATMENT OF METASTATIC BREAST CANCER WITH AMINOGLUTE-THIMIDE. R. Metz, B. Weber, J.M. Boivin

Twenty-four postmenopausal patients with metastatic breast cancer have been treated with aminoglutethimide, a potent inhibitor of adrenal steroid synthesis. Twenty of them have previously been treated with chemotherapy and/or hormonotherapy and were resistant to these drugs. The standard dose of aminoglutethimide was 250 mg four times daily, with a corticoid supplement of hydrocortisone (40 mg daily) and fludrocortisone (0.05 mg on alternate days). Six objective responses have been obtained in bone (2), lung (2), skin and peritoneal metastases, lasting from 2 to 8 months. Three of them were previously treated with tamoxifen and relapsed. In addition, five stabiliza-tions without clinical or radiological changes but with pain relief have been observed. Pain relief in bone metastases is often observed whereas the osseous lesions are in progression.
The major side-effect of the drug is a syndrome of drowsiness and lethargy, seldom dizziness or ataxia. It occurs in about 50% of patients, disappearing within a few weeks or after dose reduction for a short period. In two patients, an erythematous and morbilliform rash occurred and became very severe in one case, leading to drug interruption.

Centre A. Vautrin, Service de Médecine
54500 Vandoeuvre-les-Nancy, France

132

AZIMEXON- A NEW IMMUNOMODULATOR- IMMUNOLOGICAL AND CLINI-CAL INVESTIGATIONS. M.Micksche[1], M.Colot[1], P.Sagaster[2]

The 2-cyanaziridine analogue Imexon has already been in-vestigated by us in a phase I trial (Proc. of Conf.Immu-notherapy of Cancer - Present Status of Trials in Man, Bethesda, 1980). An analogous compound - Azimexon - has been recently developed. We have demonstrated that addi-tion of Azimexon to lymphocyte cultures in vitro enhances blastogenic response to PHA and increases percentage of active T-rosette forming cells. In animal studies we have shown that the single dose of 100 mg/kg i.p. signi-ficantly enhances spleen cell blastogenic response to PHA in vitro. In a pilot study Azimexon has been given i.v. in single doses of 200-400 mg to patients with advanced breast cancer to evaluate the effect of Azimexon during short term application (4-6 weeks) on immune function. Of 10 patients, 5 converted from negative to postive DNCB reactivity. Lymphocyte blastogenic response was also found increased after therapy. In a clinical trial (ini-tiated 1977) Azimexon is now included in an adjuvant the-rapy protocol for breast cancer. Patients are randomized after surgery to 3 treatment arms. A) No further therapy; B) Chemotherapy; C) Chemo-immunotherapy (Azimexon 1x200mg after every chemotherapy cycle). So far, 143 patients have been included in this trial.
Relapse rate is 22% in group A, 16% in group B and 9% in group C. This preliminary evaluation has to be confir-med by further follow-up and patients' input.

1. Institute for Cancer Research, Vienna University and Viennese Cooperative Study Group (I.Dept.Med.and I.Surg. Dept., Vienna University)
2. Ludwig Boltzmann Research Unit at V.Int.Dept., Wilhelminenspital, Vienna, Austria

133

PATHOLOGICAL MODIFICATIONS OF BREAST TISSUE AFTER HORMONO-CHEMOTHERAPY IN INFLAMMATORY BREAST CANCER.

L. Mignot, A.de Roquancourt , A.Gorins , D. Belpomme,
C. Gisselbrecht, M.Marty , M. Boiron

22 inflammatory breast carcinomas (18 PEV 2, 4 PEV3), were treated by an induction chemotherapy regimen including a cyclic combination of Adriamycin, 5-FU, Cyclophosphamide, Methotrexate, and Vincristine. 7 premenopausal patients received chemotherapy alone whereas 15 post-menopausal received chemotherapy + Tamoxifen. After three to four months of treatment, a mastectomy was performed followed by adjuvant hormono-chemotherapy. After induction treatment, 5 patients had a complete response and in 11 patients a tumor regression > 50 % was observed .
The overall response rate has been CR + PR = 72 %.
Initial diagnosis was obtained through needle biopsy.
(22 infiltrative poorly differentiated carcinomas).
Pathological findings were compared to those obtained after chemotherapy and surgery : they consisted of complete σ partial disorganisation of initial tumor tissue with major fibrosis particularly of the elastosis type and an increase of tumoral cell atypia.
Tumoral necrosis or inflammatory reaction was seen in two cases. In 3 patients, no neoplastic cell could be found. These aspects compared to post-radiotherapy lesions will be discussed.
Lymph nodes seemed to be less sensitive to chemotherapy than the initial tumor and no particular histological aspect could be noted. No difference was observed with or without adjunction of Tamoxifen to chemotherapy.
Histological findings will be correlated with disease free survival (median of observations 16 months).

Centre des Maladies du Sein - Unité d'Oncologie Clinique
Hôpital Saint-Louis - PARIS.

134

INTEREST OF THERMOGRAPHY IN INDUCTION HORMONO-CHEMOTHERAPY SUPERVISION FOR INFLAMMATORY BREAST CANCER.
L. Mignot, P. Sauval, R. Thierree, A. Gorins, M. Boiron.

The prognosis of inflammatory breast carcinoma is poor if treated by surgery or radiotherapy alone. There is a good correlation for prognosis between clinical inflammatory signs (PEV) and evolutive thermographical classification.
24 inflammatory breast carcinomas (PEV 2 and 3), were treated by induction hormono-chemotherapy (3 or 4 months) before local treatment (surgery or radiotherapy) followed by adjuvant medical treatment.

Initial thermography was compared with a second thermography performed at the end of induction treatment ; the thermic evolution was correlated with clinical evolution for the same period and with disease free survival (median of observation 16 months). Two thermographic signs were studied : area of hyperthermia and thermic gradient. Thermographic increase always corresponded to clinical aggravation or stabilization for local tumors. Thermic improvement (>50 %) always corresponded to partial (PR) or complete (CR) clinical response to induction treatment but clinical response (CR + PR) was observed in 70 % of all cases with a thermographic response (PR + CR) in only 58 %.
In three patients, a complete clinical and histological response was obtained but thermography still showed the same pathological aspect without recurrence after 20 months of observation.
For disease free survival, the only recurrences occurred after clinical and thermographical aggravation.
A good correlation existed between clinical and thermographical evolution whereas thermographical improvement was delayed with regards to clinical response.

Centre des Maladies du Sein - Unité d'Oncologie
Hôpital Saint-Louis - PARIS

135

CHANGES IN POLYAMINE LEVELS IN LIVER TISSUE DURING CHEMICAL HEPATOCARCINOGENESIS
G. Milano[1], C. Aussel[2], C. Stora[2], M. Lafaurie[2], M. Schneider[1], P. Cambon[1] and C.M. Lalanne[1]

During a period of 200 days, the chronological changes of polyamine levels (putrescine, spermidine, spermine) were observed in the liver of adult female Sprague Dawley rats submitted to hepatocarcinogenesis by N-2-fluorenylacetamide (FAA). Three groups of 70 rats each were used:
(1) FAA treated: 0.06% FAA in the diet; (2) control 1: low protein and low riboflavin diet; (3) control 2: normal diet.
No significant differences were noted for tissular levels of the three polyamines when the two control groups were compared. In contrast, considerable variations of these molecules were observed as a function of time in the FAA treated group: (a) an early and constant rise was seen in putrescine, with 3 maxima at days 10, 60 and 150. This last peak was the highest: 25 ± 6 nmol/g (8 times the value for the controls at this time), and coincided with the appearance of cancerous lesions. (b) while spermidine levels varied during the experiment, no significant differences were noted in comparison with the control groups. Mean levels (nmol/g) were as follows: 535 ± 108 Control 1, 552 ± 95 Control 2, 633 ± 160 FAA group. (c) spermine levels were significantly lowered, with 3 minima corresponding to the putrescine maxima. The lowest minima was observed on day 60: 114 ± 67 nmol/g, i.e. 4 times lower than the controls.
This work shows that polyamine metabolism is profoundly modified during chemical carcinogenesis, but the possible effect of polyamines on tumorigenesis itself cannot be anticipated at this point since modifications of polyamine levels are probably due to phenomena of liver necrosis and compensatory tissue proliferation observed all along the experiment.

1 Centre A. Lacassagne and 2 INSERM FRA 12 Nice, France

136

RELATIONSHIP BETWEEN POLYAMINE EXCRETION AND LABELLING INDEX IN BREAST CANCER. G. Milano, J. Gioanni, C. Azin, F. Ettore, J.-L. Boublil, M. Namer, H. Duplay, C.M.Lalanne

24-hr urinary polyamine levels were measured for 34 patients with primary breast cancer just prior to tumor surgery. The labelling index (LI) was evaluated on tumor tissue fragments from the surgical specimen. Polyamines (putrescine PU, spermidine SPD) were quantified by ion exchange on an automatic amino acid analyzer (KONTRON, Liqquimat III). Patient ages ranged from 33 to 83 (mean 59). Values of the various study parameters were: PU (µg/mg of creatinine), $\bar{m}$ 2.13, limits 0.73-4.60, normal upper limit of healthy controls ($\bar{m}$ + 2 SD, n=22) = 2.00; SPD (µg/mg creat.), $\bar{m}$ 1.59, limits 0.46-4.00, normal upper limit of healthy controls ($\bar{m}$ + 2 SD, n=22) = 1.60; LI $\bar{m}$ = 2.72 %, limits 0-6.80.
Correlation coefficients between LI and polyamines were both positive but not significant: PU/LI r = 0.30; SPD/LI r = 0.26. Of interest is the fact that low LI values (0-2%, n=16) were associated with 81% of low PU levels (<2 µg/mg creat., 13 of 16); high LI values (>2%, n=18) were linked to 72% of elevated PU levels (>2 µg/mg creat., 13 of 18) (p < 0.01). No such association was found between LI and SPD.
While various animal experiments have demonstrated a direct relationship between polyamine levels and tumor growth rate, in vivo human proofs are needed to validate clinical research for polyamines in cancer. These results, based on a specific in vivo human study, demonstrate the existence of a good association between urinary PU and LI in breast cancer. This emphasizes the notion that PU reflects cellular proliferation and, consequently, that polyamines may be considered markers of tumor kinetics when measured in biological fluids from cancer patients.

Centre Antoine Lacassagne, 36 Voie Romaine
06054 Nice Cédex, France

137

LYMPHOBLASTIC LYMPHOMA (LYMPHOSARCOMA).
J.L. Misset, F. Calvo, D. Pontvert, D. Belpomme & G. Mathé

Lymphoblastic lymphoma (LL) can be recognized as a clinicopathologic entity. The cells which are of intermediate size
and not hyperbasophilic can be distinguished from those of
Burkitt's tumor but not from those of acute leukemias. Mi-
toses are frequent.
Since 1976 we have treated 19 patients with LL without bone
marrow involvement at presentation. The disease arises predominantly in children and young adults under 30 years of
age, but a few cases were seen in older patients (pts.).
10 pts. became leukemic in the course of the disease. These patients were compared with 24 pts. diagnosed as leukemic lymphoma at referral, differing from acute lymphoblastic leukemia by important involvement of organs other than
lymphoid organs contrasting with bone marrow involvement
which is only partial. Natural history of the two groups
of patients was identical, thus allowing to consider them
as having the same disease which we call "lymphoblastic
lymphoma or lymphosarcoma". Prognostic factors were studied within this group of 43 pts. Age has no influence on
prognosis nor has stage or initial involvement of bone
marrow. Mediastinal involvement is a highly predictive
prognostic factor, 75% of the patients without this involvement being alive at 30 months vs. 28% of the pts. with
mediastinal presentation.
Similarly, immunologic markers were predictive of prognosis: 75% of the pts. with "null cell" type were alive at
30 months and the median survival time was 50 months, while it was only 14 months for the pts. with T-cell lymphoblastic disease who all died within 15 months.
Those two factors are only partially linked.

Hôpital Paul-Brousse, Institut de Cancérologie et
d'Immunogénétique, 94800-VILLEJUIF (France).

138

NEUROPROPHYLAXIS IN ACUTE LYMPHOBLASTIC LEUKEMIA. CORRELA-
TION OF NEUROLOGICAL RISK AND EFFICACY OF PREVENTION WITH
OTHER PROGNOSTIC FACTORS. J.L. Misset, F. De Vassal,
Cl. Jasmin and G. Mathé.

252 patients with acute lymphoblastic leukemia (ALL) have
been retrospectively reviewed for neurological involvement
(N.I.) and prophylaxis. In a historical group of 76 patients who received no CNS prophylaxis or less than 5 intrathecal (I.T.) injections of methotrexate (MTX), 26 patients
(34%) had N.I. as first site of relapse (F.S.R.). 69 Patients received craniospinal irradiation (1,000 to 1,500 rads)
plus 12 to 18 I.T. injections of MTX with or without cytosine arabinoside. Only 5 patients (7%) had N.I. as F.S.R.
The last group of 107 patients received cranial irradiation (2,400 rads) plus 8 to 12 I.T. injections of MTX. The
same incidence of N.I. was seen: 10/107 (9%) as F.S.R.
Thus, no difference appears in terms of efficiency between
the 2 modalities of neuroprophylaxis.
Moreover, 136 patients of the last 2 groups could be stratified according to prognostic criteria described elsewhere[+]
According to these criteria, only one case of N.I. as F.S.
R. was observed in the good prognosis group of 52 patients
whether given 1,000 to 1,500 rads + I.T. injections (inj.)
(0/22) or 2,400 rads + I.T. inj. (1/30), while 11 cases of
N.I. as F.S.R. were observed in the poor prognosis group
of 84 patients (15%) regardless of the prophylaxis given:
in the 1,000 to 1,500 rads group, 4/26 patients (15%); in
the 2,400 rads group, 9/58 patients (15%). We therefore
think that neuromeningeal risk is not identical in prognostic subclasses of ALL. The prophylaxis routinely given
today is very efficient in good prognosis subgroup and may
even be too aggressive if various complications recently
described are taken into account, while optimal prophylaxis
remains to be defined in poor risk patients.

[+] Medical and Pediatric Oncology, 4, 17-27, (1978).

Hôpital Paul Brousse, Institut de Cancérologie et
d'Immunogénétique, 94800-VILLEJUIF (France).

139

CENTROFOLLICULAR SMALL OR LARGE NON-IMMUNOBLASTIC CELL
LYMPHOMA.
J.L. Misset, M. Gil-Delgado, M. Delgado and G. Mathé

Centrofollicular lymphoma (CF L) can be recognized as a
clinicopathologic entity. Histologically it can be nodular
or diffuse. The constitutive cells have a wide range of size and on Giemsa stained smears or imprints appear intermediate between the small lymphocyte and the lymphoblast.
Cytoplasm is not hyperbasophilic as that of immunoblasts.
On immunologic studies, they are almost always monoclonal
B-cells. Since 1976 we have collected 121 patients (pts.)
with such defined CF L. Age distribution is similar to that
of chronic lymphoid leukemia, with virtually no children,
and a frequency peak between 40 and 60 years of age. At
referral time 50 pts. were at stage III and 55 pts. at
stage IV. 50 had nodular L and 68 diffuse L (3 unclassi-
fied). 70 pts. had predominantly small cell L and 51 had
predominantly large cell L, the two factors being linked
(only 8 pts. with large cell nodular L) (p $<$ 0,001). Stage
III and IV patients, previously untreated, received combined modality therapy including induction chemotherapy with
adriamycin, VM26, cytoxan and prednisone, radiotherapy on
icebergs, complementary chemotherapy by vincristine, cytoxan and prednisone (CVP). Patients who arrived in first
complete remission at the end of this program were randomized to receive, or not, immunotherapy with BCG. Stage I &
II patients were given CVP after radiotherapy. Survival
was 60% at five years. Prognostic factors were mainly histological patterns with an 85% five year survival for the
nodular group vs. 40% for the diffuse group (p $<$ 0,001).
Predominant cell size was even more predictive of prognosis with 85% pts. surviving at 5 years in the small cell
group and 25% pts. surviving at 5 years in the large cell
subgroup (p $< 10^{-6}$).
On the whole centrofollicular L appears to be of better
prognosis than lymphoblastic and immunoblastic L.

Hôpital Paul-Brousse, Institut de Cancérologie et
d'Immunogénétique, 94800-VILLEJUIF (France).

140

CLINICAL AND IMMUNOLOGICAL EXPERIENCE OF INTERFERON IN
B-CELL MALIGNANCIES. J.L. Misset, A. Goutner & G. Mathé

Seven patients with B-cell chronic lymphocytic leukemia
(CLL) were treated with human leukocyte interferon (Pasteur Institute, Paris). Treatment consisted of 10 day pulses of 25,000 to 100,000 units/kg s.c. each day with intervals of 10 to 20 days between each course and dose escalation in the same patient whenever possible. Side effects were frequent for high dosages (100,000 U/kg) and
consisted of chills, fever, malaise. Biological tolerance
was good.
Peripheral lymphocytosis was significantly decreased in
five patients out of seven patients, sometimes temporarily. Lymph node or spleen enlargement was significantly decreased in only one instance. In one patient leukemic skin
involvement completely disappeared. In all cases, NK cell
activity was significantly enhanced and this enhancement
was not dose related and was transient.
Three additional patients with CLL have been treated by
continuous daily administration of 1.5 million s.c. for
three months. One patient progressed, the two others being
in good partial remission with no side effects. NK cell
activity is also transiently enhanced with this schedule.
10 patients with myeloma (nine IGG - one IGA) were treated
with human fibroblastic interferon (R.P.M.I. Buffalo). The
schedule was 3.10^6 U I.V. every three days for 45 days,
the dose being escalated to 3.10^6 each day for another 45 days in the absence of response. Anaphylactic reactions required treatment discontinuation in two instances;
side effects were otherwise comparable to those of human
leukocyte interferon. Antitumor activity was observed in
some cases, relief of pain in 3 out of 4 patients, decrease of M component in 3 patients, decrease in plasma cell
bone marrow infiltration in 3 patients.

Hôpital Paul-Brousse : Institut de Cancérologie et
d'Immunogénétique, 94800-VILLEJUIF (France).

141

CONTINUOUS INFUSION ADRIAMYCIN: RATIONALE AND PRELIMINARY
RESULTS. F. Muggia, M. Levin, J. Wernz, J. Bottino,
R. Blum and J. Speyer

Acute gastrointestinal intolerance and other symptoms including cardiac arrhythmias complicate treatment with
adriamycin. This has encouraged the use of regimens em-
ploying amounts which have less than optimal efficacy.
In addition, the risk of heart disease leads to avoidance
of adriamycin in conditions such as sarcomas, or breast,
endometrial, bladder and prostatic carcinomas of the el-
derly even when it may be potentially beneficial.
Initial experience by the MD Anderson Hospital indicates
modification of acute toxicities by infusion adriamcyin
(Legha et al., Proc. AACR & ASCO, 1979) and also dimin-
ished cardiotoxicity (Benjamin et al, unpublished).
Accordingly the administration of adriamycin by 24 hr continuous infusion in high flow venous systems has been
initiated at NYU. The design has been of a Phase I/II
study with initial doses of 60 mg/m^2 escalating to 75
mg/m^2 and to 90 mg/m^2 if nadir counts were WBC $\geq$ 3,000
and platelets $\geq$ 100,000. 22 patients have been entered
with an age range from 30 to 79 and a median of 56. Results of these studies show that the infusions are well
tolerated and toxicities including nausea and mucositis
are minimal or absent. Pharmacologic data and study of
resting and exercise ejection fractions by radionuclide
gated pool scans are ongoing. The recommended starting
doses for a Phase II trial are 60 mg/m^2 for previously
treated or poor risk patients and 75 mg/m^2 for untreated
patients. An occasional patient tolerates 90 mg/m^2 with
minimal hematologic change. Therapeutic effects have
been noted in a patient with breast cancer who had previously progressed on lower bolus doses of adriamycin,
in a patient with cervical cancer and in 2 patients with
endometrial cancer, ages 79 and 56. Phase II trials
are continuing in lung and endometrial cancer.

New York University Cancer Center, Division of Oncology
550 First Avenue, New York, NY 10016

142

PROGNOSTIC FACTORS IN METASTASED BREAST CANCER.M.Namer,J.L.
Boublil,M.Abbes,M.Hery,M.Francoual,J.L.Moll,C.M.Lalanne

Numerous studies to define prognostic factors for breast
cancer patients have recently added the presence or not of
hormone receptors and histological grading to the already
recognized parameters of tumor size and number of axillary
nodes involved. These 4 parameters are used to define
groups with different risks of metastasis and thus different survival curves. Our study was aimed at determining
whether all patients who   later metastased regardless of
their initial classification conserved their initial prognostic differences or whether the occurence of metastases
annulled initial particularities. 78 patients who had relapsed after breast cancer were classed according to primary tumor characteristics (tumor size, presence or not of
metastased axillary nodes) and relapse-related parameters
(estradiol receptors, histological grade). Distribution of
these prognostic factors for these patients was compared
with the distribution of the same factors for breast cancer patients for whom the outcome was unknown. Survival
curves, free intervals, and evolution under treatment were
also studied and results grouped according to prognostic
factors. Results : prognostic factors continue to influence
survival and response to therapy even after metastases have
occurred. Survival rates at 5 years were : 54% for T1/T2;
24% for T3/T4; 67% for R+; 30% for R-; 79% for N-; 13% for
N1-2-3 (all percentages statistically significant). 3/15
patients have died in the group of all patients with the
best prognostic factors (T1/T2, R+) whereas only 3/15 patients were still alive after 5 years in the group of all
those with the worst prognosis (T3/T4, R-). Prognostic factors linked to the primary tumor thus continue to influence disease evolution, even when all patients with metastases are classed together and even if relapse occurs long
after the primary tumor. These 4 prognostic factors thus
well individualize tumor types with differing doubling times, a characteristic which persists all along the course
of the disease.

Centre Antoine-Lacassagne,36 Voie Romaine,06054 NICE Cedex

143

PHASE II STUDY OF CIS-DICHLORODIAMMINEPLATINUM (II) (DDP)
IN OESOPHAGOEAL SQUAMOUS CELL CARCINOMA (O.S.C.C.).
S. Nasca, P. Coninx, S. Segal, R. Brossel, E. Boulenger,
A. Cattan

A prospective study was carried out to determine the effectiveness of DDP (100 mg/sq. m.) given i.v., with hydration and mannitol infusion, every 3 weeks to patients
with measurable or evaluable lesions of primary or metastatic O.S.C.C. Between March 1978 and May 1980, 18 patients with histologically documented tumours entered the
study. Among those patients, 13 had metastatic disease
whereas the five others had a localized tumour. Nine patients had received previous treatment : chemotherapy (1)
and radiotherapy (8). Among 9 evaluable primary tumours,
one complete and one minor regression were observed. In
ten patients with pulmonary metastases, two minor, two
partial and two complete regressions (in one case for 24$^+$
months) were achieved. In 6 patients with involved lymph
nodes, 5 partial and 1 complete regression were obtained.
Assessment of the overall response in each patient was
based on the lesion with the smallest regression. The
pattern of responders was as follows : 3 C.R. ; 2 P.R. ;
3 minor R. The over-all response rate was therefore 44 %
(8/18). This chemotherapy was reasonably well-tolerated.
The number of courses given to each patient varied from
2 to 6. There was no lethal toxicity but the treatment
had to be stopped in two cases for renal, auditive and
cerebral (?) impairment. Although other toxic effects
were common and nearly constant such as vomiting, they
were mild to moderate. Briefly, DDP treatment resulted in
an overall response rate of 44 % with mild toxicity. Accordingly, that would be the most effective drug in O.S.
C.C.

Institut Jean-Godinot - B.P. 171 - 51056 REIMS Cédex.

144

PILOT STUDY OF THIAZOLIDINE-4-CARBOXYLIC ACID (THIOPROLI-
NE) IN THE TREATMENT OF ADVANCED TUMOURS. S. Nasca,
V. Galichet, P. Coninx, A. Cattan

A prospective study was achieved with thioproline to determine its effectiveness and tolerance in patients with
measurable or evaluable lesions of advanced tumours. Thioproline was given daily in 4 equal doses according to one
of 3 schedules : a) oral administration (20 mg/kg/d) for
at least 3 weeks ; b) i.m. administration (40 mg/kg/d) as
sodium salt for at least 2 weeks ; c) as b), but for a
week every 3 weeks. From March 1980 to June 1980, 48 patients with histologically documented tumours entered the
study. 22 patients on the first schedule have been receiving thioproline for a median time of 45 days (21 to 92 d)
11 were bearing squamous cell carcinoma whereas the others
were suffering from adenocarcinoma. One half of those patients had received previous treatment. 9 men on the second schedule have been receiving thioproline for head and
neck cancer for a median time of 29 days (9 to 42 d.). 5
patients out of them had not been treated previously. Until now, 17 patients on the third schedule have received
between 1 to 3 courses. Among them, there were 8 tumours
classified as squamous cell carcinoma. Whatever the schedule no one regression was observed even in well differentiated squamous cell carcinoma. On the contrary, some toxic effects were exhibited. Of the 22 patients on the
first schedule, 4 got moderate disturbances in the renal
function where as 3 others suffered from cerebral impairment and one had both manifestations. Among 9 patients on
the second schedule, 5 demonstrated the same renal side
effects and 3 of them had cerebral manifestations simultaneously. Until now, no side effects which resulted from
third schedule appeared at all. In conclusion, this study
does not confirm the previous hopeful results in the treatment of squamous cell carcinoma.

Institut Jean-Godinot - B.P. 171 - 51056 REIMS Cédex.

145

THE TREATMENT OF OSTEOSARCOMA WITH INTERFERON AND LOCAL TUMOUR RESECTION, Nilsonne, U.

Interferon is a physiological antiviral substance produced by all cells infected by viruses. In in vitro systems interferon also has shown inhibitory effects on tumour cells, which has particularly been demonstrated in osteosarcoma cell lines in our laboratory. Since 1972 interferon has been given to a consecutive series of osteosarcoma patients without signs of metastases at the time of admission to the hospital. Interferon is given as intramuscular injections as adjuvant therapy for 1.5 years. The surgery consists of local tumour resection, followed by reconstruction by endoprosthesis or bone grafting. In cases with extensive tumour growth ablative surgery has to be resorted to. Irradiation was only given to a few patients at the start of the series and chemotherapy was not used at all. The present five-year survival achieved is 50%. In 35% of the cases local surgery instead of amputation was performed.

Dept. of Orthopaedic Surgery, Karolinska Hospital
Stockholm, Sweden.

146

CYTOTOXIC AUTOREACTIVE CELLS, THEIR POSSIBLE ROLE IN SYNGENEIC BONE MARROW TRANSPLANTATION.

L. Olsson, N. Kiger and G. Mathé

Cytotoxic autoreactive cells (CAuC) with natural killer cell-like function have been demonstrated to have an important antineoplastic effect in several murine tumor systems. A monoclonal antibody with high specificity to CAuC has been used to demonstrate the existence of CAuC in various organs in normal mice. By isolating CAuC with fluorescence-activated cell sorting, it has further been shown that such cells may influence take-frequency of otherwise syngeneic bone marrow grafts. These cells may also induce a wasting-like syndrome by grafting to syngeneic recipients. The importance of similar human CAuC on human bone marrow transplantation is discussed.

ICIG, Hôpital Paul-Brousse, F-94800 Villejuif, France

147

MEDICAL ADRENALECTOMY WITH AMINOGLUTETHIMIDE-CORTISOL IN ADVANCED BREAST CANCER : CLINICAL RESULTS AND FACTORS INFLUENCING RESPONSE. R.Paridaens, J.C.Heuson

Fifty-three post-menopausal patients with recurrent metastatic or locally advanced inoperable breast carcinoma were treated in a phase II trial with Aminoglutethimide (1.0 g/day) plus low-dose cortisol replacement therapy(40mg/day) Treatment was stopped rapidly because of intolerance in 7 patients. Thirty-nine were evaluable and response was assessed according to UICC criteria. Fifteen patients (38.5%) displayed an objective partial response (2 to 19 months) and 13 are still in remission. Nine patients had a mixed response (2 cases) or stabilization (7 cases) (3+ to 21 months). Treatment failure with early neoplastic progression occurred in 15 patients (38.5%). Several factors were analyzed as to their putative predictive value with regard to response. High estrogen receptor concentrations (ER $\geqslant$ 100 fmoles/mg tissue protein) were associated with a high proportion of responses (4/5; 80%) whereas no remission occurred in six cases with lower ER concentrations. Other favorable prognostic factors were a long disease-free interval, increasing age and increasing number of years after the menopause. Response rates by site were the following : soft tissue 13/24 (54%); bone 6/25 (24%); viscera 4/16 (25%, mainly lung or pleural metastases). These results are comparable to those reported by other groups using higher doses of corticosteroids. Side effects occurred in 27/53 patients (51%) and consisted generally of skin rashes and drowsiness appearing early in the course of therapy. A low initial dosage of Aminoglutethimide (500 mg/day) allowed reduction of the incidence and severity of these complications. Signs of adrenal insufficiency were never observed after cessation of treatment. Medical adrenalectomy is an effective endocrine treatment for postmenopausal patients with advanced breast cancer. It can be proposed as first-line treatment in cases with presumably hormone-dependent tumors.

Serv.Méd., Clin.et Lab.Cancérol.Mam.,Inst.J.Bordet, rue Héger-Bordet,1, 1000 Brussels, Belgium.

148

PHASE II TRIAL WITH N-(PHOSPHONOACETYL)-L-ASPARTATE (PALA) IN ADVANCED BREAST CANCER. R.Paridaens, JC Heuson, T. Palshof, M. Mouridsen, E.Engelsman, H.Cortes-Funes, J. Michel, S.Ciatto, J.Vermorken,N.Rotmensz and M.Rozencweig.

PALA is a synthetic antimetabolite with anticancer activity in a variety of murine solid tumors including the C3H mammary carcinoma and the human mammary xenograft MX-1. Thirty-nine eligible patients with far advanced breast cancer were entered in this phase II clinical trial.Of 30 patients who went off study, 2 were lost to follow-up and 4 were early deaths. Response was evaluated in 24 women with a median age of 57 yrs (32-72) and a median performance status of 80(60-100).All had been previously treated with radiotherapy, chemotherapy and hormonotherapy.Visceral disease was present in 12 patients. Pretreatment characteristics also included WBC >3,000/mm3,platelets > 75,000/mm3,creatinine ≤ 1.2 mg/dl and bilirubin <1.5mg/dl. PALA was given as a 60-min iv infusion at a daily dose of 2.5 g/m2 for 2 consecutive days.Courses were repeated every 2 weeks.The study protocol called for dose escalations when no toxicity was encountered.The median number of courses per patient was 3 (2-10). Two patients achieved partial response (>50%) for 4.5 and 3 months from initiation of therapy. These patients had soft tissue and visceral dominant disease respectively. Five patients had unchanged disease after 5 to 9 courses of PALA.Drug-induced toxic effects were evaluated in 28 patients.Mucocutaneous toxicity was most frequently encountered with skin toxicity (13pts), stomatitis (13pts), diarrhea (12pts), conjunctivitis (3pts), corneal ulceration (2pts) and vaginitis (1pt). Other side-effects included nausea-vomiting (13pts) dizziness or somnolence (4 pts) and hypotension (1pt). Apparently drug-related leukopenia (WBC <4000/mm3) was noted in 2 courses among patients with WBC >4000/mm3 upon entry into the trial. These preliminary results in far advanced disease suggest that PALA might be an effective drug against breast cancer. This drug deserves consideration for combination chemotherapy in this disease.

EORTC Breast Cancer Cooperative Group.

149

DIRECT CLONING OF HUMAN MALIGNANT TUMORS IN SOFT AGAR.
Pavelic, Z.P., Slocum, H.K., Nowak, N.J. and Rustum, Y.M.
Direct cloning of neoplasms in semisolid cultures has potential for a) predicting responses to anticancer agents,b)
screening of new oncolytic compounds and c) clarification
of tumor biology. This study describes the results from
158 human solid tumors and 6 non-neoplastic tissue specimens taken directly from 155 patients and set up in agar.
Cells were disaggregated by enzymatic method consisting of
microtome slicing of tissues and incubation at 37°C for 2
hr in RPMI 1640 medium containing 10% fetal calf serum 0.8%
collagenase II, and 0.002 deoxyribonuclease I(Slocum et al,
AACR, 21:187,1980). Tumor cells were cultured in a 2-
layer agar system (0.5% agar feeder, 0.3% plating layer)in
enriched medium without adding conditioned medium. Colonies were defined to be aggregates of >30 cells and clusters as aggregates of 5 to 30 cells. Colony size varied
from 30 cells to greater than 1000 cells and the time to
maximal growth varied from 10 to 30 days. The number of
colonies from 5 x 10^5 cells ranged from 50 to 16,000 per
plate, yielding plating efficiency from 0.01 to 3.2%. Considerable variations in plating efficiency were noticed
between individual tumors of the same type. Ninety of 158
malignant tumors (20/33 melanoma, 14/33 lung carcinoma,
18/27 sarcoma, 11/15 colon carcinoma, 9/18 breast carcinoma, 6/7 ovarian carcinoma and 12/25 other solid tumors)
were successfully grown in the soft agar system yielding
an overall cloning incidence of 57%. Contamination of
tissue cultures was found in 12% of cases, mostly in lung
and breast carcinoma. A linear relationship was obtained
between the number of cells plated and the number of colonies. Morphological characteristics of tumor cells forming the colonies in agar were similar to those of tumor
cells in the original cell suspension. The histological
pattern of the original tumors was maintained after passage from agar-methyl cellulose into the nude mouse. (Supported by USPHS Grants CA-21071, CA-24538 and CA-13038).

Roswell Park Memorial Institute, Buffalo, New York 14263,
U.S.A.

150

LEVAMISOLE THERAPY DURING MAINTENANCE OF REMISSION IN
PATIENTS WITH ACUTE LYMPHOBLASTIC LEUKEMIA. S. Pavlovsky,
G. Garay, F. Sackmann Muriel, E. Svarch and GATLA, Buenos
Aires, Argentina.

Two groups of patients with acute lymphoblastic
leukemia (ALL) treated with two consecutive protocols and
in their first complete remission (CR) were randomized to
receive or not levamisole (LEV). All the variables of both
protocols in intensification, maintenance, CNS prevention
or reinforcement pulses were similar to   each other
in the duration of CR. LEV was given at 120 mg/m2/d po.
No difference emerges in prognostic parameters of age and
WBC count at diagnosis between the LEV and the control
group. Twenty-nine out of 146 children with good risk
(<50000 WBC count) treated with LEV had bone marrow
relapse compared to 50 out of 147 in the control group,
69% and 52% respectively remain in remission at 48 months
(P<0.001). Seventeen out of 39 patients with high risk
(<15 years and >50000 WBC count and adults) had bone
marrow relapse and 37 out of 61 in the control group; 43%
and 23% remain in remission at 36 months (P=N.S.). Eight
(4%) out of 185 patients treated with LEV died in CR and
21 (10%) out of 208 in the control group (P<0.05). A total
of 47% and 33% of all the patients with and without LEV
remain free of disease (without CNS, marrow or testes
relapse) and are alive at 48 months (P<0.0005). Survival
since diagnosis was, in good risk, at 60 months, 60% in
the LEV group and 35% in the control group (P<0.0005).
In high risk, at 48 months, 34% and 33% respectively
(P=N.S.). We conclude that LEV used as adjuvant of
maintenance chemotherapy significantly prolongs the
duration of hematological remission and survival of ALL
patients with good risk.

Dr. Santiago Pavlovsky, Instituto de Investigaciones Hema
tológicas, Oncohematology Dept., P. de Melo 3081, Buenos
Aires, Argentina.

151

PHASE I CLINICAL TRIAL WITH ANTHRACENEDIONE DIACETATE
(DAD)(NSC-287513). M. Piccart, M. Rozencweig, R. Abele,
E. Cumps and Y. Kenis.

DAD is a new aminoanthraquinone derivative that achieves
antitumor activity in a large variety of animal models.It
is a dark blue dye. In this phase I study, the drug was
given as a 30-min iv infusion repeated every 3 weeks.Nine-
teen patients were entered in the trial and received a total of 43 courses. All were adult patients with advanced
solid tumors, mainly squamous cell carcinoma of the head
and neck and malignant melanoma. Sixteen had prior chemotherapy and only 1 had not been previously treated. Median age was 56 yrs (39-74) and median performance status
was 70 (40-90). None of the patients treated with toxic
doses had bilirubin >1.5 mg% or creatinine >1.5 mg%. The
trial was initiated at a starting dose of 10 mg/m2 and
dose levels were escalated up to 180 mg/m2.Leukopenia was
dose-related, well predictable, reversible and dose-limiting. At 135 mg/m2, the median WBC nadir was 1,800 (1,100-
4,400) and the median PMN nadir was 948 (460-2,244).Among
all courses, WBC nadir occurred on median day 12 (8-18)
and recovery was seen on median day 16 (10-29). Thrombocytopenia (<100,000) was encountered in 2 courses. There
was no evidence of cumulative myelosuppression with repeated courses. Non-hematological toxic effects were negligible and included stomatitis in 1 course,minor alopecia in 3 patients, questionably drug-related orthostatic
hypotension in 3 patients. Reversible green-blue skin
discoloration was seen in 5 patients at 75 (1), 135 (2)
and 180 mg/m2 (2). All patients treated with >40 mg/m2
had dark blue urines for 2 or 3 days. Nonspecific transient EKG changes were noted in 2 patients. Antitumor activity with response >50% could not be documented.In conclusion, DAD appears to be very well tolerated and easy
to handle. Its clinical anticancer potential remains to
be determined. A dose-schedule of 135 mg/m2 q 3 weeks may
be recommended for phase II studies in solid tumors.

Institut Jules Bordet, Brussels.

152

ALPHA NAPHTYL ACETATE ESTERASE AND PEROXIDASE ACTIVITY
IN HUMAN AUTOLOGOUS ROSETTE FORMING CELLS (ARFC).
P.Philip*, J.F.Quaranta*; M.Schneider;*R.Masseyeff*.

Non-specific esterases and peroxidases have been
considered as markers for discriminating monocytes and
macrophages from lymphocytes. Acid alpha naphtyl acetate
esterase (ANAE) is now considered as a marker for human
T cells. However, null cells also show esterase activity
but in the form of multiple spots like in most Fc γ T cells
instead of the single spot observed in Fc μ T cells and in
a few Fc γ T cells, or generalized granular cytoplasmic
activity in monocytes-macrophages. In this work, autologous rosettes which are formed by a T cell subpopulation
have been stained in smears for peroxidase and ANAE. No
peroxidase activity was observed. Conversely, scattered
granules of ANAE were seen in most ARFC. It is generally
agreed that this scattered pattern of ANAE is found in T
cells bearing Fc γ receptors and in Con A activated cells.
The Fc γ T cells have been demonstrated to be also "activated" cells. Thus, most ARFC may be also interpreted as
activated T cells. The fact that ANAE show two different
cellular distributions may be related to a hypothetical
function of this enzyme in the cytotoxic or amplifying
(lymphokine like) effect of ARFC.
*   INSERM FRA I2, Laboratoire d'Immunologie du CHU,
    06034 NICE Cedex.
** Laboratoire d'Hématologie-Cancérologie, Centre Antoine
    Lacassagne, 06054 NICE Cedex.

153

DISSEMINATED BREAST CARCINOMA/ PRELIMINARY RESULTS OF A
RANDOMIZED TRIAL COMPARING THE THERAPEUTIC EFFECTIVENESS
OF CHEMOTHERAPY TO CHEMOTHERAPY PLUS TAMOXIFEN AND TO
CHEMOTHERAPY PLUS TAMOXIFEN AND A PROGESTOGEN.
P. Pouillart, M. Jouve, T. Palangie, E. Garcia-Giralt,
H. Magdelenat, B. Asselain

159 patients with histologically proven disseminated
breast cancer entered this trial from October 1978 to
October 1979: 59 patients in group I received a monthly
course of combination chemotherapy including: Adriamycin
(40 mg/m2, on day 1) + Cyclophosphamide (400 mg/day, on
days 2,3,4) + 5-Fluorouracil (500 mg/m2, on days 2,3,4).
54 patients in group II were given the same combination
chemotherapy and daily administration of 30 mg tamoxifen.
46 patients in group III received the same combination
chemotherapy and daily administration of 30 mg tamoxifen
plus 60 mg Norethisterone.
An objective response was observed in 31 patients in
group I (61%), in 45 of group II (80%) and in 37 from
group III (80%). The difference between group I and
groups II and III is highly significant: $X 2 = 53.6$,
$p < 0.0001$. Comparison of actuarial survival curves
showed a significant difference in favor of groups II and
III (p : 0.03), but no difference appears in survival
between group II and group III. The analysis of results
stratified according to the level of hormone receptors in
the tumors showed that survival was comparable in patients
with oestrogen receptors (p : 0.84), but the presence of
progesterone receptors has a very high prognostic significance (p : 0.005).

Service de Médecine Oncologique, Institut Curie
26 rue d'Ulm, 75231 Paris Cédex 05, France

154

ADVANCED OVARIAN CARCINOMA. RESULTS OF A COMBINATION
CHEMOTHERAPY WITH ADRIAMYCIN, CYCLOPHOSPHAMIDE, 5 FLUO-
ROURACIL ASSOCIATED OR NOT WITH CIS DDP. P.Pouillart,
T.Palangié, B.Bretaudeau, E.Garcia-Giralt, B.Asselain

56 patients with ovarian carcinoma, stade III and IV entered this trial. 23 patients in group I were given a
monthly course of a combination chemotherapy with Adriamycin : 40 mg/m2 on day 1; Cyclophosphamide : 400 mg/m2
on days 2-3-4 and 5 Fluorouracil : 600 mg/m2 on days
2-3-4. 17 patients in group II (never treated before)
were treated according the same program plus Cis DDP :
60 mg/m2 on day 4; 16 patients in group III were in relapse after chemotherapy and were treated with the same
regimen as used in group II. Toxicity was moderately severe : nephrotoxicity was observed in 1 patient in group
II; hypoplasia developed in 2 patients in group III who
died from infectious complications.
In group I, 14 patients (61%) had objective partial (7)
or complete (7) remissions for a projected median duration of 10 months. In group II, 11 patients (65%) had
objective partial (6) or complete (5) remissions. In
group III, 7 patients had objective partial (3) or complete (4) responses. The median of survival is over 17
months for patients of groups I and II and of 14 months
for patients of group III.
An analysis of major prognostic factors will be presented.

Service de Médecine Oncologique, Institut Curie,
26 rue d'Ulm, 75231 Paris Cedex 05, France

155

ADVANCED BREAST CARCINOMA. RESULTS OF PILOT TRIAL OF IN-
TENSIVE AND AMBULATORY CHEMOTHERAPY PROGRAM INCLUDING :
ADRIAMYCIN, MITOMYCINE C, CYCLOPHOSPHAMIDE AND METHOTRE-
XATE. P.Pouillart, T.Palangié, M.Jouve, E.Garcia-Giralt

63 patients were included in the pilot trial: 20 patients
presented an inflammatory breast carcinoma (group I) : 10
patients an advanced breast tumor considered as T4 N3
(group II); 27 patients metastatic breast cancer (group
III) and 6 patients an inflammatory local relapse after
radiation therapy (group IV).These patients were given a
segmential combination chemotherapy including : Adriamycin
: 45mg/m2 on day 1; Cyclophosphamide : 600 mg/m2 on days
1 and 23; Methotrexate : 20 mg/m2 on days 2-9-24-31; Mitomycine C : 10 mg/m2 on day 23. The courses of treatment
were repeated every 45 days. After 3 complete courses of
treatment a cumulative hematological toxicity with predominant anemia appeared in 70% of the patients and 2 patients in group III have developed acute severe pancyto-
penia. Alopecia was present in 90% of the patients after
3 courses of treatment; mild stomatitis was noted in 35%
of the cases. In group I : 5 patients had a complete response or a partial (>50%) and 5 a partial (<50%) response.
In group II, 1 patient had a complete response and 7 a
partial response. In group III, 9 patients had a complete
response and 21 a partial response. In group IV, 9 patients
had a complete response and 2 a partial response. The
overall results showed a complete response in 12/63 (19%)
or partial (>50%) response in 28/63 (44%), a partial
(<50%) response in 18/63 (29%), a total failure in 5/63
(8%). This intensive combination chemotherapy seems to be
a good candidate for induction therapy for locally advanced tumors as inflammatory breast cancer.

Institut Curie, Service de Médecine Oncologique,
26 rue d'Ulm, 75231 Paris Cedex 05, France

156

COMBINATION OF 5 FLUOROURACIL, MITOMYCINE C, CYTOSINE
ARABINOSIDE AND CIS DDP IN ADVANCED COLORECTAL CARCI-
NOMAS. RESULTS OF A PHASE II TRIAL. P.Pouillart ,T.
Palangie ,M.Jouve,E.Garcia-Giralt

16 patients with advanced colorectal carcinomas entered   this trial from May 1979 to May 1980. The chemotherapy was administered in patients who presented no
visceral failure and when creatininea was under 110µ/l
The chemotherapy regimen included : -5 Fluorouracil :
600 mg/m2/day on days 1-2-3, in a 2 hours IV infusion;
-Mitomycine C : 10 mg/m2 on day 1 in IV injection ;
-Cytosine Arabinoside : 240 mg/m2 on day 2, in 24
hours IV infusion ;- Cis DDP : 80 mg/m2 on day 2, in
a 2 hour IV infusion. The courses of treatment were
repeated every month. The digestive tolerance was
nausea and vomiting were observed in all the cases.
Diarrhea appeared in 11 patients 2 to 6 hours after
Cis DDP infusion and   persisted for 6 to 8 hours.
A renal toxicity with transient elevation of creatininemia was observed in 2 cases after 3 courses of treatment ; these complications led us to stop the chemotherapy. In 1 patient   deafness appeared after 5
courses of treatment. The hematological tolerance was
generally acceptable during the first 6 months. 1 patient presented a transient but severe manifestation
of hypoplasia with infectious complications. After 4
to 6 courses of chemotherapy, cumulative and delayed
hematological toxicity probably related to Mitomycine
C administration led us to increase the interval between courses of treatment. Objective response over
50 % lasting 3 to+12 months was obtained in 5 patients and a minor response in 5 other patients. 3
patients did not respond to treatment and in 3 patients   stabilisation was obtained for 3 months. No
relation between sites of tumors and sensitivity to
treatment was observed.
Service de Médecine Oncologique.
Institut Curie, 26, rue d'Ulm, 75231 Paris Cedex 05

40

157

SURVIVAL OF PATIENTS WITH METASTATIC BREAST CANCER
TREATED WITH ENDOCRINE OR CHEMOTHERAPY. T.J. Powles.

Overall survival of patients with breast cancer has
not improved in spite of increasing use of multiple
drug chemotherapy for patients with metastases.
Although objective regression of tumour occurs in
70% of patients with metastases there is no evidence
that there is improved overall survival from first
relapse of patients given multiple drug chemotherapy.

We have compared survival from first relapse of 100
patients given a combination of Vincrisine, Adriamycin
and prednisolone (VAP) in a phase II study with 100
patients given Aminoglutethimide in a similar phase II
study. Although responders to VAP survived significantly better than non-responders, patients who
responded to Aminoglutethimide (or had stabilisation
of disease) survived best of all. Furthermore, all
patients given Aminoglutethimide survived better
than those given VAP.   There is no doubt that many
patients given VAP had improved survival and/or
palliation.

These results indicate the need to identify those
patients who benefit from chemotherapy. There is also
a need to attempt to improve the response rate to
endocrine therapy.

Royal Marsden Hospital, Department of Medicine,
Downs Road, Sutton, Surrey, U.K.

158

MULTIPLE ENDOCRINE THERAPY FOR TREATMENT OF METASTATIC
BREAST CANCER. A PHASE III STUDY. T.J. Powles, R.C.
Coombes.

Tamoxifen, Aminoglutethimide and Danazol are hormones
shown to cause objective regression of tumour deposits
in patients with metastatic breast cancer. Each has
a response rate of approximately 30% but they all
probably act on different cytoplasmic receptors.
Furthermore, the type of patients and site of metastases
are somewhat different for responders to each type of
treatment. We have, therefore, compared the response
rate and survival of patients given a combination of
Tamoxifen 10 mg.b.d., Aminoglutethimide 250 mg t.d.s.,
and Danazol 100 mg. t.d.s. with patients given only
Tamoxifen 10 mg.b.d. and subsequently given the other
hormones if indicated, in a randomised clinical trial.

So far, 77 patients have been randomised into the Trial
and the early results indicate a similar response rate.
Larger and more accurate results will be available in
the next three months.

Royal Marsden Hospital, Department of Medicine,
Downs Road, Sutton, Surrey, U.K.

159

PROGNOSTIC VALUE OF LYMPHOIS DIFFERENTIATION MARKERS IN
B-CELL NON-HODGKIN LYMPHOMA. E. Pujade-Lauraine+,
D. Belpomme++, M. Henri-Amar+++, B. Caillou+++,
A.J.S. Davies++++, G. Mathé+++++

Human lymphoid neoplasias are thought to be frozen at
various stages of cell maturation. Study of malignant
cells of 145 cases of non-Hodgkin lymphomas (NHL) with
respect to several characteristics known to change
sequentially during normal lymphoid differentiation
(1) immunological membrane markers; (2) cell size;
(3) tissue distribution; (4) pattern of growth, has
allowed us to separate B-cell NHL into four distinct
groups. Evidence is brought that these four groups are
associated with different clinical presentation and prognosis, suggesting a correlation between prognosis and
malignant cell differentiation in B-cell NHL. The value
of individualization of these four groups, which favors
in several points the W.H.O. classification, will be
discussed in comparison with the other currently used
histo-cytological classifications.

+   Hôpital Beaujon, Clichy, France (Prof P. Boivin)
++   Hôpital St Louis, Paris, France (Prof M Boiron)
+++   Institut Gustave Roussy, Villejuif, France
++++ Chester Beatty Research Institute, London, U.K.
+++++ ICIG, Hôpital Paul Brousse, Villejuif, France

160

CHEMOTHERAPY OF ADVANCED EXTRAGONADAL GERM CELL TUMORS
WITH CISPLATIN, VINBLASTINE AND BLEOMYCIN. R. Quiben,
C. Mendiola, M. Mendez, A. Manas, H. Cortés Funes

Twelve patients with advanced extragonadal germ cell
tumors were treated with a PVB combination at doses and
on a scheme reported previously (Proc. Euro. Soc. Med.
Oncol., 53, p. 14, 1979). The primary was located in the
mediastinum in 11 patients and 1 was sacrocoxigeal.
There were 6 embryonal carcinomas (4 mixed), 2 malignant
teratomas and 4 seminomas. Three patients had been
previously treated with chemotherapy or radiotherapy.
All were evaluable for response and toxicity. Overall
response was 83.3% with 6/12 CR (50%) and 4/12 PR.
Two of these partial responses were under treatment for
a residual mediastinal mass after 3 cycles of chemotherapy. All seminoma patients responded to treatment.
Neither of the previously treated patients achieved CR.
Toxicity was mild, with one treatment-related death.
From this data we can conclude that: (1) extragonadal
germ cell tumors are the same as gonadal germ cell tumors
with a different location, with a lower CR rate; and
(2) primary mediastinal seminomas are very sensitive
to the PVB regimen and chemotherapy must be considered
an ideal treatment in such cases.

Seccion de Oncologia Médica,
Hospital "1° de Octubre"
Madrid, Spain

161

BIOCHEMICAL MARKERS RELATED TO SURVIVAL IN GASTRIC
CANCER. S.A. Rashid, J. O'Quigley, E.H. Cooper and the
Yorkshire Gastrointestinal Cancer Group.

Serum carcinoembryonic antigen (Pharmacia PRIST) and
α_1-antichymotrypsin (ACT) (Behringwerke)   were measured
pre-operatively in 105 patients with gastric cancer.
Patients in whom both levels were raised (25) had a
median survival of 5 weeks; those with normal levels(32),
>91 weeks and those with only one abnormal parameter(48)
had a median survival of 20 weeks.

Statistical analysis, using a regression model, showed
that these pre-operative measurements could add
information relating to prognosis even when operative
and histological findings were taken into account.

To validate our initial results a further prospective
study of stomach cancer is now in progress with 50
patients accrued to date.   The general applicability
of this predictive system and the inter-relationships
of the clinical and biochemical factors and survival
will be presented.

Unit for Cancer Research, University of Leeds, England.

162

STAGING AND PROGNOSIS IN ACUTE MYELOID LEUKEMIA
(AML). P. Reizenstein, B. Andersson, N. Giannou-
lis, R. Hast, B. Nordenskjöld, L. Skoog, B. Tho-
rell

Several reports indicate limited prognostic use
of morphologic, FAB-classification of AML. History provides better prognosis; 1-year survival
was 45% of 58 AML patients at first diagnosis
under 60 years and without preleukemia, versus
5% of older patients, or those with preleukemia
(p<0.01). To further classify the younger patients, functional cellular characteristics were
studied. In the patients under 60 years, 14-month
survival is 72% if they have neither >50 cellclo-
nes in peripheral blood agar cultures (CFU_c), nor
>25% immune response-like antigen (Ia) positive
cells, nor more than 1000 ng ferritin/ml serum,
nor more than 95% blast cells in the differential
count at diagnosis. In patients who have one or
more of these signs, 14 month survival is only
22% (p<0.05). Alternatively, the presence of corticosteroid receptors can be used. In patients
whose leukemic cells have receptors over 0.25
fmol/ug DNA, 6 month survival is 88%, versus 10%
in those whose cells have less corticosteroid
receptor content (p<0.01).

P. Reizenstein, Div. of Hematology, Dept. of Medicine, Karolinska Hospital, S-104 01 STOCKHOLM,
Sweden.

163

EVALUATION OF DIBROMODULCITOL IN ADVANCED MALIGNANT
MELANOMA. A PHASE II STUDY. S.Retsas, T.Mughal, K.A.Newton,
G.Westbury

Twenty patients with advanced malignant melanoma resistant
to or relapsing from previous cytotoxic chemotherapy were
admitted to a phase II study for the evaluation of the
anti-tumour activity of Dibromodulcitol.
The drug was given orally in one of two schedules :
1) 10 mg/kg of body weight as a single dose every 5 days
or 2) 100 mg/m^2 of body surface area as a single dose
daily, in the evenings. Both schedules were continued until haematologic toxicity ensued. Eight patients are not
considered evaluable because of inadequate treatment with
the drug (total dose <3 G). Of the twelve evaluable patients all had previously received vindesine, 11 had received DTIC and three various other drugs including m-AMSA
Nine patients had advanced visceral metastases and in
three cutaneous disease only was detectable. The median
duration of treatment was 6 weeks (range 3-22). The median
total dose of Dibromodulcitol was 5.4 G (range 3-14 G).
Nine patients experienced a more than 50% reduction of
WBCs and or platelets during therapy compared to pretreatment values. Leukopenia and thromocytopenia were recovera-
ble on withdrawal of the drug.
No objective regressions were observed. The disease sta-
bilized clinically in three patients for periods ranging
from three to six months. Two of these patients had extensive liver deposits with ascites in one, and a third had
cutaneous lesions only. Tolerance to the drug was excellent. Although objective regressions of visceral metastases have been reported with Dibromodulcitol in resistant
malignant melanoma, we are so far unable to confirm this
experience with the present study.

Westminster Hospital, London SW1, United Kingdom

164

IN VITRO AND IN VIVO EVALUATION OF LEVAMISOLE IN RENAL
ADENOCARCINOMA. S.Retsas, C.Thomas, K.A.Newton, J.R.Hobbs
The mixed lymphocyte reaction in culture (MLR) of 21 patients with renal adenocarcinoma was studied, without and
with levamisole, added in eight different molar concentrations and was compared with that of 22 normal volunteers.
The MLR of patients did not improve when levamisole was
added to the cultures in molar concentrations ranging from
10^{-9} to 10^{-2}. Almost identical results were obtained from
the study of lymphocytes of the 22 normal controls :

	MLR (mean counts per minute)			
	No levamisole		optimal MLR with Lev.	
Patients	18051	N.S.D.	17646	(10^{-3})
Controls	55190	N.S.D.	52397	(10^{-5})

Seventeen patients from the same group, 12 with stage IV
and 5 with clinical stage III disease received levamisole
in a dose of 2.5-3 mg/kg of body weight on two consecutive
days every week, for periods ranging from one month to two
years. Drug tolerance in this group of patients has been
discussed elsewhere (Retsas et al., the Lancet,1978,pp 324-
325). No objective responses were seen. With one excention
disease progressed while the patients were on levamisole
therapy. This drug was stopped after two years treatment
in one patient with stage III disease who 12 months later
developed pulmonary metastases. The immune profile of
seven patients was evaluated at monthly intervals with the
MLR and absolute blood lymphocyte counts while they received levamisole for periods ranging from six to fourteen
months. An observed trend of improvement of the MLR in
some cases during treatment did not correlate with disease
inactivity. There is no in vitro evidence supporting the
value of Levamisole therapy in renal adenocarcinoma and
the clinical results of a pilot study in this group of
patients tend to support this.

Westminster Hospital, London SW1, United Kingdom

165

TREATMENT OF MALIGNANT NON-HODGKIN'S LYMPHOMAS WITH FAVORABLE HISTOLOGY BY AN ASSOCIATION OF POLYCHEMOTHERAPY AND TOTAL BODY IRRADIATION (TBI). Results of a pilot study. P. Richaud, G. Hœrni-Simon, G. Denépoux, M. Durand, B. Hœrni, C. Lagarde

Sixteen patients with malignant non-Hodgkin's lymphomas with favorable histology were treated by an association of radio + chemotherapy. The patients were classified stage III or IV after a radioclinical work-up without surgical investigation. Induction polychemotherapy (C.V.P.A.) consisted of one course of an association with adriamycin (35mg/m2 on day I and 15), vincristine (0.7mg/m2 on day 1, 8 and 15), cyclophosphamide (400 mg/m2 on day 1, 8 and 15) and prednisone (40mg/m2 from day 1 to day 14). Afterwards the patients received monochemotherapy for six weeks in order to allow bone marrow recovery before (TBI). Irradiation consisted of two series of 0.75 Gy in 5 fractions on 5 consecutive days with 2 weeks interval of rest. Lastly, after an interval of 4 weeks, the patient again received a course of chemotherapy identical to the first one (C.V.P.A.).

This protocol was well tolerated, easy to carry out, reproducible and did not burden the patients. Its immediate efficacy (15 complete remissions achieved in 16 patients) and good tolerance have incited us to carry out further long term studies on a larger number of patients and to compare these results to chemotherapy alone or TBI alone.

Fondation Bergonié, 180 rue de Saint Genès, F33076 Bordeaux Cédex

166

PHARMACOKINETICS OF ADRIAMYCIN (ADM) IN PATIENTS WITH BREAST CANCER : CORRELATION BETWEEN PHARMACOKINETIC PARAMETERS AND CLINICAL SHORT-TERM RESPONSE. J. Robert, B. Hœrni and M. Durand.

The pharmacokinetics of adriamycin was evaluated in the plasma of 11 patients with breast cancer after injection of an IV bolus. The patients (mean age : 55 ys) suffered from a locally advanced tumor with inflammatory signs and were free of hepatic metastases. They received a combined chemotherapy consisting of ADM (50 mg/m^2) on day 1, vincristine (1 mg/m^2) on day 2 and methotrexate (6 mg/m^2) on days 3, 4 and 5. The response to chemotherapy was assessed as the percent of reduction of the palpable tumor mass 3 weeks after the first course of chemotherapy. Plasma samples were collected at various times after injection of the drug. ADM and its metabolites were extracted using an original column purification technique and were evaluated by HPLC with fluorometric detection. Pharmacokinetic parameters were calculated based on a three compartment model by successive linear regression analysis of the decay curve obtained by semi-logarithmic plotting. The three successive half-lives were 5.63 $\pm$ 1.1 min, 70 $\pm$ 32 min and 21.3 $\pm$ 4.2 h. The maximal interindividual ratio obtained was 1 : 2.5. The volumes of the three compartments were in contrast highly different from one patient to another and the maximal interindividual ratio was 1 : 9. The total plasma clearance of the parent drug ranged from 217 to 1282 ml/mn No correlation was found between either of the three half-lives and the clinical response ; however, significant negative correlations were observed between the volumes of the compartments or the total plasmatic clearance and the clinical response. We can therefore assume that the short-term efficacy of the drug is dependent upon its distribution in the organism. Such a relationship may allow the development of new protocols of chemotherapy in order to obtain an optimal distribution of the drug in every patient.

Fondation Bergonié, 180 rue de Saint-Genès, 33 BORDEAUX.

167

PROSTAGLANDIN SYNTHESIS AND CELLULAR AUTONOMY IN HUMAN BREAST CANCER. P.H.Rolland, P.M.Martin

Synthesis of prostaglandin (PG) occurs in a number of malignant tumors. Yet little is known about the production and biological significance of PG in cancer. We have previously presented evidence suggesting that an elevated PG production is a marker of high metastatic potential for neoplastic cells. To further examine the properties of PG producing cells, PG production in each lesion of a representative population of breast tumors was related to size and clinical extension, histological features (histologic type HT and differentiation HD, and histoprognostic grade HPG) and hormone status (steroid receptor SR content). PG production was elevated in tumors having a limited extent as graded (T-classification) by IUAC. PG production was low in differentiated and/or low HPG carcinomas, and elevated in carcinomas that retained a minute part of the acino-ductal differentiation and in tumors with a moderate degree of cancer. Thereafter, PG production decreases in tumors of large extent, in undifferentiated lesions and in cancers w/ a high HGP value. Consequently, PG production decreases in 3 different situations in which an active tumor spread has or is still occurring : a) as the tumor grows; b) as acino-ductal differentiation drops, and c) as cancer degree increases in lesions. Concerning SR which are proposed to reflect hormone and tissular dependence of human breast cancer, we now report that a lesion containing SR produced less PG than did an SR negative. In contrast, a relationship could be established between PG production and cellular autonomy, i.e. the loss of the host-tissue component relationships of reciprocal dependence.
From these results, we propose that the high metastatic potential of PG producing neoplastic cells is due to the improvement of the cellular autonomy which is concomitant with loss of tissular dependence for these cells.

Laboratoire des Récepteurs Hormonaux, Faculté de Médecine de Marseille(secteur Nord), 13326 Marseille Cedex 3,France

168

PREOPERATIVE CHEMOTHERAPY OF LOCALLY ADVANCED BREAST CARCINOMA (INFLAMMATORY TYPE). G. Rosset, P. Alberto, F. Krauer

The poor prognosis of inflammatory type breast carcinoma (described as PEV II and III) may be linked to the high frequency of undetected micrometastases at the time of diagnosis leading to frequent and rapid dissemination of the disease. It seems of interest to combine early general chemotherapy with local treatment.
We have treated 14 patients (7 premenopausal, 7 postmenopausal) with the following chemotherapy schedule: Adriamycin 6 mg/m2 on days 1 and 8; Chlorambucil 5 mg/m2 on days 1 to 14; Methotrexate 10 mg/m2 IV on days 1 and 8 and Fluorouracil 500 mg/m2 IV on days 1 and 8. The same treatment was repeated monthly for 2 to 6 cycles depending on clinical results.
Modified radical mastectomy was then performed. Response rate to chemotherapy with complete clinical remission was obtained in 11 cases, but the histological examination showed persistence of numerous malignant cells in the mastectomy specimens. Tolerance was good, leading to no surgical complications. Post-operative follow-up will be discussed.

This pilot study was supported by the Swiss Group (SAKK).

Hôpital Cantonal, 1211 Geneva 4, Switzerland

169

MEDULLARY THYROID CARCINOMA. IMPORTANCE OF CALCITONIN AND CARCINOEMBRYONIC ANTIGEN MEASUREMENT. Ph Rougier, C. Calmette, C. Parmentier, G. Milhaud, M. Tubiana

Serum calcitonin (CT) is a good marker of medullary thyroid carcinoma (MTC) and for a decade has been used in its diagnosis ; more recently it was found that carcinoembryonic antigen (CEA) also is a reliable marker. Our aim was to evaluate the prognostic value of both markers on a retrospective study of 27 patients treated at Villejuif.Twelve of them were assessed before and after initial treatment. Out of them in 3 patients CT came back to a normal level after a complete surgical excision and in the 9 others CT level remained higher than normal, 4 of these 9 patients had had an incomplete treatment (3 metastases and 1 important cervical extension),the 5 remaining had had an apparently satisfactory surgical treatment. Six of the 8 patients having had   satisfactory surgical treatment had cervical lymph node involvement, only in 1 of them CT level fell to a normal level. In 15 other patients the first CT assay was performed only a few months after initial treatment. Out of the 27 patients for whom post treatment CT level was available,8 had been incompletely treated,their CT and CEA were higher than those of the 19 patients in complete remission after treatment, 4 of these 8 patients deceased rapidly.Nineteen patients were in complete remission,out of them 8 had a normal CT level and all remained free of disease with a mean follow-up of 7.5 years (0.6 to 11 years);11 patients in complete remission had a high CT level,3 of them relapsed. All these 11 patients had initially   lymph node involvement; furthermore in 9 of them the surgical excision had been difficult.
No patient with abnormal CT level had a normal CEA level. Three to 9 months after treatment CEA level does not appear to predict recurrence better than does CT level.However, for 2 of the 27 patients CEA has been a more reliable marker of the course of disease. Furthermore,all patients who recurred had had a high CEA level.

Service de Médecine Nucléaire, Institut Gustave-Roussy, 94800 VILLEJUIF, et Hôpital Saint Antoine 75012 PARIS

170

CISPLATIN IN REFRACTORY TUMORS-A PHASE II STUDY R.B. Schilcher,M.Scheulen,N.Niederle,C.G.Schmidt

Seventy patients with refractory, progressive solid tumors of different histologies were entered into a phase II-study of cisplatin (DDP). The dosage was 2o mg/m^2 days 1-5 iv q 3 weeks. Ten patients who failed on this low dose DDP protocol received   intermittent high dose therapy (DDP 1oo mg/m^2 over 6 hours iv q 2-3 weeks; hydration and forced diureses).
In sixty-seven evaluable patients, there were 4 CR (malignant melanoma, spindle cell sarcoma, adrenal carcinoma, bladder carcinoma), in 24 patients (36%) a PR was obtained, 19 patients (28%) showed NC and 2o (29%) had tumor progression. A response rate of 33% (4/12 patients) was seen in malignant melanoma, 42% (3/7) in bronchogenic carcinoma-3/4 patients with large cell carcinoma had a PR-and 42% (6/14) in sarcomas of various types. The responses lasted from 1 to 9 months, median 2 months.
The ten patients treated with high dose DDP (melanoma n=2, terato carcinomas of the testes n=5, sarcoma n=2 and Hodgkin's disease n=1) received between 1 and 5 courses; in 6 patients NC was obtained; 4 other patients had continuously progressive tumors.
Although the therapeutic effect of DDP was short lived in this unfavourable patient selection, the high response rates especially in patients with malignant melanoma, bronchogenic carcinoma and sarcoma, refractory to conventional chemotherapy, justify the incorporation of DDP into combination chemotherapy programs in these tumors. The data also indicate that high dose intermittent DDP may be marginally superior to the low dose regimen.

Innere Universitätsklinik (Tumorforschung) West German Tumor Center, D 43oo Essen, FRG

171

SEQUENTIAL COMBINATION CHEMOTHERAPY WITH VINBLASTINE/BLEO-MYCIN AND ADRIAMYCIN/CIS-DICHLORODIAMMINEPLATINUM (II) IN NON-SEMINOMATOUS TESTICULAR CANCER
I. Results of a prospective randomized phase III study with 71 patients with disseminated disease (stage IV) C.G. Schmidt

74 patients with disseminated non-seminomatous testicular cancer were randomly entered on a prospective sequential combination chemotherapy regimen with mandatory crossover consisting of either Vinblastine/Bleomycin or Adriamycin/ Cis-dichlorodiammineplatinum (II) (DDP) as initial therapy Independent of the randomization, the overall remission rate in 71 evaluable patients was 89%, including 54% complete remissions. 35% of the patients remained disease-free at 2+ to 28+ months (median 12 months). By additional surgical removal of residual pulmonary metastases in 2 patients, the complete remission rate was increased to 40/71 (56%), and the number of patients with no evidence of disease to 27/71 (38%). According to the life-table method, the 2-year survival rates were 63% for complete responders and 29% for all other patients, which was significantly lower. 53 patients (75%) were alive at 3 to 28 months (median 9 months). Additional advanced abdominal disease, initially elevated β-HCG and LDH and extension of pulmonary disease were of significant negative influence on the prognosis. The evaluation of single chemotherapy courses revealed equal efficacy of both combinations. However, response to Adriamycin/DDP occurred in 46% of the courses when Vinblastine/Bleomycin had failed, while response to Vinblastine/Bleomycin occurred in only 21% of the courses when Adriamycin/DDP had failed. Thus, different patterns of cross-resistance may exist between these alternative regimens.

Prof. Dr. C.G. Schmidt
Innere Universitäts-u. Poliklinik (Tumorforschung)
West German Tumor Center
Hufelandstrasse 55, 4300 Essen, West Germany

172

SEQUENTIAL COMBINATION CHEMOTHERAPY WITH VINBLASTINE/BLEOMYCIN AND ADRIAMYCIN/CIS-DICHLORODIAMMINEPLATINUM (II) IN NON-SEMINOMATOUS TESTICULAR CANCER

II. LONG-TERM RESULTS OF A STUDY WITH 140 PATIENTS WITH RETROPERITONEAL DISEASE (STAGE II) C. G. Schmidt

Following orchiectomy and retroperitoneal lymph node dissection (RND) 140 patients with stage II non-seminomatous testicular cancer were treated by sequential combination chemotherapy consisting of Vinblastine/Bleomycin and Adriamycin/cis-dichlorodiammineplatinum (II) (DDP), plus/minus radiotherapy. 68 stage IIA-patients (complete RND and normal tumor-markers thereafter) received 6 courses of chemotherapy, followed by radiotherapy in 35 patients. 40 stage IIB-patients (minor residual disease after RND or elevated tumor-markers after RND) and 32 stage IIC-patients (advanced residual disease after RND) were treated by at least 12 chemotherapy courses and optional intermittent radiotherapy and/or relaparotomy. In stage IIA and IIB disease the actuarial 4-year survival rates were between 80 and 100 %. These favourable results were not significantly influenced by additional radiotherapy and corresponded to the survival rates for 34 stage I patients. For stage IIC patients the prognosis was significantly worse with a 12% 4-year survival rate.

Prof. Dr. C.G.Schmidt
Innere Universitäts-u. Poliklinik
(Tumorforschung)
West German Tumor Center
Hufelandstr. 55   43oo Essen

173

SELECTION OF PATIENTS WITH COLORECTAL ADENOCARCINOMAS SUITABLE FOR ADJUVANT CHEMOTHERAPY WITH 5FU AND BCNU BY THE NUDE MOUSE TESTING MODEL. R.Schmitz, W.Nikolaizik, C.Gerdts, C.Seidler

In order to determine the individual response of primarily xenotransplanted human adenocarcinomas to 5FU and BCNU, 20 different colorectal human adenocarcinomas were treated with a combination of 5FU (8 mg/kg BW) and BCNU (175 mg/m²) after growth on collectives of syngeneic, female BALB/c-nude mice. The tumor take was about 82% in the mean. The method of transplantation and documentation of tissue remission was carried out as described by the author earlier. Humnan adenocarcinomas of stages DUKES A and B (n=6) were followed by strong initial remissions and a continuing volume decrease after xenotransplantation and treatment. DUKES C and (D) tumors showed no tumor remission compared to untreated controls. Pathohistologically, the tumors responsive to therapy showed a strong tendency to necrosis up to 50%, while non-responsive tumors had necrosis up to 20%/tumor only. The results show that histologically identical human colorectal adenocarcinomas differ in their individual response to the same 5FU and BCNU chemotherapy, which depends on the tumor staging. Patients with adenocarcinomas of stages DUKES A and B should be subjected to post-operative chemotherapy with BCNU and 5FU with a prospect of success.

Klinik für Abdominal-und Transplantationschirurgie der Medizinischen Hochschule Hannover. Karl-Wiechert-Allee 9, D-3000 Hannover, FRG.

174

IMMUNORESTORATIVE PROPERTIES OF AZIMEXON
L. Schwarzenberg, A. Goutner and G. Mathé

Immunodepression is very frequent in cancer patients, resulting from presence of a tumour or as a consequence of chemotherapy or radiotherapy. We have studied the immunorestorative properties of azimexon, a new synthetic immunoadjuvant. 11/16 anergic cancer patients bearing various solid tumours have experienced a restoration of their delayed type hypersensitivity reactions after receiving per os 200mg of azimexon per day, 3 days/week, for 2 weeks. No toxicity has been observed with this dosage. In addition, 7 out of 9 breast cancer patients without tumour but immunodepressed after chemotherapy and/or radiotherapy have been restored by azimexon. In vitro studies in these two categories of patients have shown that azimexon acts on the functional properties of a T lymphocyte population with high affinity receptors for sheep red blood cells and responding to the selective mitogen tetradecanoyl phorbol acetate (TPA), and enhance the cytotoxic activity of the natural killer cells against K562 target cells in a ^{51}chromium release assay.

Thus, azimexon is able to restore delayed type hypersensitivity reactivity and to stimulate spontaneous cell mediated cytotoxicity. Azimexon is now studied in phase III trials.

Hôpital Paul-Brousse : Institut de Cancérologie et d'Immunogénètique (INSERM U-50), 94800-Villejuif, France.

175

EFFICACY OF A BENZAMIDE DERIVATIVE IN THE PREVENTION OF NAUSEA AND VOMITING DUE TO CHEMOTHERAPY. B. Serrou, D. Cupissol, F. Favier

The efficacy of two new anti-emetic drugs, the oxoglurate of di-arginine (Eucol) and a benzamide derivative (SL 7906) was tested in two groups of 20 cancer patients treated by chemotherapy. These two groups were compared to a matched control group of 20 cancer patients treated with the same chemotherapy in which metoclopramide (Primperan) and metopimazine (Vogalene) were used as anti-emetic drugs. The chemotherapy drugs injected IV were Adriamycin, Cyclophosphamide, 5-FU, DTIC and CDDP. All of these patients prior to this study had experienced nausea and vomiting during the chemotherapy treatment. Eucol was administered IV at a dose of 30 g per day. 10 mg of benzamide derivative were injected intratubularly at the beginning of the chemotherapy treatment; 10 mg were added to the serum perfusion given during the antimitotic treatment. Primperan and Vogalene were injected as previously described for the latter drug. There was no significant difference between Vogalene and Primperan as compared to Eucol. However, liver function tests and chemotherapy tolerance were better with Eucol. A significant decrease (p < 0.05) in vomiting was observed with the benzamide derivative, especially in patients treated by CDDP. Sleepiness was also observed in 9 patients who received this benzamide derivative.

Laboratoire d'Immunopharmacologie des Tumeurs FRA-INSERM n° 46; ERA-CNRS n° 844 and Dept. of Chemo-Immunotherapy C.R.L.C., B.P. 5054, 34033 Montpellier Cêdex, France

176

PHASE I STUDY OF A RETINOIC ACID DERIVATIVE IN CANCER PATIENTS. B. Serrou, D. Cupissol, F. Favier

Solid tumor bearing patients are often immunodepressed, and this immunodepression may be increased by the chemotherapy treatment. A reasonable approach would therefore consist of immunorestauration and/or immunostimulation before and after chemotherapy. The immunorestorative effect of a retinoic acid derivative was evaluated as a function of auto-rosette forming cells (ARFC) and delayed hypersensitivity skin tests (Mérieux system) before and after treatment (5 mg/kg/P.O. of retinoic acid derivative for 15 days) in 28 patients with advanced solid tumors. Patient distribution was: 13 breast cancers, 7 digestive tract cancers, and 8 malignant melanomas. The age of patients ranged from 42 to 67. The results show a significant increase in ARFC from 12.5 to 15.7% (p < 0.001) and a significant improvement for delayed hypersensitivity skin tests (Mérieux score 8.11 cm to 20.8 cm; p < 0.02). Two minor skin rashes, but no major side-effects, were observed during this treatment.

Laboratoire d'Immunopharmacologie des Tumeurs FRA-INSERM n° 46; ERA-CNRS n° 844 and Dept. of Chemo-Immunotherapy, C.R.L.C., B.P. 5054, 34033 Montpellier Cêdex, France

177

PHASE I ONGOING STUDY OF BESTATIN IN PATIENTS BEARING
ADVANCED SOLID TUMORS. B. Serrou+, D. Cupissol, H. Flad,
A. Goutner, J.M. Lang, H. Spirzglas, R. Plagne, M. Beltzer
P. Chollet, J.C. Petit, G. Mathé

Previous work has clearly demonstrated that the median
survival is much improved in patients in whom immunity
was restored to normal levels. For these reasons, we
evaluated the immunorestorative potential of Bestatin.
In vivo, the immunorestorative properties of Bestatin were
evaluated as a function of delayed hypersensitivity skin
tests (Mérieux system), auto-rosette forming cell (ARFC)
level, and NK activity before and after treatment (40 mg
three times a week for two weeks P.O.) in 29 patients
with advanced and metastased solid tumors. The results
show a significant increase in ARFC and NK activity
($p < 0.05$) and a clear improvement for the delayed hypersensitivity skin tests (Mérieux score: $p < 0.05$). In
one patient who took a one month dose all at one time, a
cutaneous rash was noted. In 20 other patients followed
for 6 months, no major side-effects were observed. Furthermore, in 3 patients with a high number of ARFC before
treatment we observed a clear drop after two weeks of
treatment, suggesting that Bestatin can modulate the
immune response depending on the immune status at the
beginning of treatment.

EORTC Cancer Immunology and Immunotherapy Group
+ Laboratoire d'Immunopharmacologie des Tumeurs FRA-INSERM
  n° 46; ERA-CNRS n° 844 and Dept. of Chemo-Immunotherapy
  C.R.L.C., B.P. 5054, 34033 Montpellier Cédex, France

178

TOWARD QUALITATIVE ARTIFICIAL NUTRITION IN CANCER PATIENTS
B. Serrou+, D. Cupissol+, C. Rosenfeld++
Quantitative artificial peripheral intravenous alimenta-
tion (APIA) defined by the number of kcal a day given to
patients, is widely used as an adjunct cancer treatment.
However, it is expensive and no clear evidence has been
brought for its efficacy. In a non-randomized but matched
trial conducted on patients presenting advanced solid tumors resistant to chemotherapy (epidermoid cancers and digestive tract tumors), we have shown that APIA significantly increases the response rate to chemotherapy and
certain immunological parameters as compared with the
matched group. In a second randomized study with patients
bearing oat cell carcinoma treated by chemotherapy, we
have not found any significant advantage for the group
receiving APIA as an adjunct treatment. These results,
and discrepancies reported in the literature, suggested
to us that APIA could improve patient status but might
also, in certain conditions, enhance tumor growth. Furthermore, recent data emphasized tha fact that it could
be possible to manipulate tumor growth, at least in ani-
man models, and the immune response by acting at the
level of nutrients (lipids, amino acids, zinc, vitamins,
insulin, etc.). Our results and these data prompted us to
evaluate the role of lipids in the host-tumor relationship. We have been able to show (1) increased microvis-
cosity in patients bearing advanced solid tumors, (2)
20% intralipids (widely used in APIA) given in vivo can
decrease the number of circulating auto-rosette forming
cells and modulate local tumor growth and the appearance
of lung metastases in mice tumor systems. Such preliminary results suggest cautious utilization of APIA in
cancer patients.

+Laboratoire d'Immunopharmacologie des Tumeurs FRA-INSERM
n° 46 - ERA-CNRS n° 844 & Dept. of Chemo-immunotherapy,
CRLC, B.P. 5054, 34033 Montpellier Cédex, France
++ ICIG, Hôpital Paul Brousse, 14-16 av. P.V. Couturier,
94800 Villejuif, France

179

IMMUNIZATION AGAINST MURINE MELANOMA W/ B-16 MELANOMA CELLS
TREATED WITH VIBRIO-CHOLERAE-NEURAMINIDASE (N'ase).
M.Shafir, J.F.Holland, J.G.Bekesi

In an attempt to evaluate the therapeutic effectiveness
of VCN'ase treated B-16 melanoma cells, 8-10 week old
male $C_{57}B1$ mice were immunized subcutaneously (s.c.) or
intra-cranially (i.c.) with tumor vaccine. Four groups of
mice were used : a) (s.c.) immunization, b)(i.c.) immunization, c) sham immunization (s.c.) and d) sham immunization (i.c.). The immunogenicity of B-16 melanoma in $C_{57}B1$
mice was significantly increased after treatment with VCN'
ase.$C_{57}B1$ mice immunized (s.c.) with VCN'ase treated tumor cells rejected subsequent challenge of 10^5 untreated
melanoma cells, which is approximately 10^3 times the LD_{50}
for this tumor. Sera and splenic lymphocytes from the immunized (s.c.) $C_{57}B1$ mice neutralized the tumorigenicity
of B-16 melanoma and protected the recipient $C_{57}B1$ mice
against the disease. Immune lymphocytes pretreated with
anti-θ sera lost this ability to neutralize the tumorigenicity of B-16 melanoma. In the (i.c.) control group all
animals died between 6 and 12 days after (i.c.) challenge.
Mice immunized (i.c.) with VCN'ase treated melanoma cells
and subsequently challenged with 10^5 untreated melanoma
cells (i.c.) showed an increase in survival to 19.4 days,
$p > .003$. This indicates therapeutic effectiveness of (i.c.)
administered VCN'ase treated tumor vaccine and suggests
that the central nervous system is not immunologically inert.

Mount Sinai School of Medicine, Fifth Avenue and 100th
Street, New York, N.Y. 10029, USA.

Supported by NCI Special Virus Contract #/NO1 CP 43225

180

SMALL CELL CARCINOMA OF LUNG, LONG TERM RESULTS OF COM-
BINED TREATMENT. M. R. Shetty, J. W. Brouhard, B. S.
Devi, S. Stefani, R. K. Arora
23 patients with small cell lung cancer were treated
from 3/76 to 7/80 with chemotherapy and radiation therapy.
There were 17 males and 6 females. 10 patients had
limited disease and 13 patients had extensive disease.
Ages ranged from 33 to 68 years. Radiation therapy
(R.T.) was delivered to primary tumor and regional
nodes (4500 r to 5000 r in 5 weeks) and prophylactically
to the brain (2500 r to 3000 r in 10 fractions). Concomitant chemotherapy with Cytoxan (750 mg./M^2) was
given every 3 weeks. Upon completion of R.T., Vincristine (1.4 mg./M^2) Adriamycin (50 mg./M^2) were added to
Cytoxan. After cumulative dose of Adriamycin to
550 mg./M^2, Cytoxan was continued as maintenance therapy.
Toxicity was nausea, vomiting and alopecia. Myelosuppression was not a problem. 11 patients lived from 10
to 45 months. 3 patients developed central nervous
system relapses. In 5 patients the tumor size was
3 cm. 3 of these are alive and free of disease at 27,
31 and 52 months. 1 lived 30 months and 1 patient 10
months. 2 of the 3 living patients had pneumonectomy
and a lobectomy. 8 of 23 patients lived 1 year. 4 of
23 lived 2 years. Tumor size of <3 cm. and surgery
have important roles in producing long term survival.

Northwest Community Hospital, 800 West Central Road,
Arlington Heights, Illinois, 60005.

46

181

BIOSYNTHESIS OF AN ANTIINFLAMMATORY FEEDBACK MEDIATOR
IN MALIGNANT TUMOURS.
K.W. Stahl, I. Vergnon, G. Mathé

On the basis of a semiquantitative test using murine
peritoneal macrophages as an analytical tool (1) the
biosynthesis of an antiinflammatory , phagotoxic (2)
antikinin peptide (3) has been studied:
Antikinin production in vitro needs the presence of both
serum and malignant cells. The synthesis is markedly increased in the presence of the di-isopropylfluorophosphate
(DIFP) inactivated molecular weight fraction 10^4-10^5 of
fetal calf serum (FCS). When, however, tumour cells are
exposed to 1 mM DIFP or 100 ug/ml N-α-p-Tosyl-1-Lysine
Chloromethyl Ketone HCL (TLCK) for 15 min at room temperature washed twice and then incubated with FCS, antikinin
formation is inhibited almost completely.
From this it may be concluded that antikinin biosynthesis
needs a macromolecular precursor which can be furnished
by serum and a protease seeping from or secreted by
malignant cells. Antikinin appears to be a negative feedback mediator responsible for the local inhibition of
an inflammatory reaction in destructively invading
tumours.

This work is part of a project (I 35/040)
sponsored by the STIFTUNG VOLKSWAGENWERK

1. STAHL, K.-W. et al. (1980) Fresenius Z. Anal. Chem.
   301, 196
2. FAUVE, R.M. et al. (1974) Proc. Nat. Acad. Sci. USA
   71, 4052 - 4056
3. STAHL, K.-W. et al. (1977) in Proc. EURES Symposium
   "The Macrophage and Cancer", 271 -280

I.C.I.G., U. 50 INSERM
F-94800 Villejuif, France

182

SHIPBUILDING ASSOCIATED MESOTHELIOMA IN COASTAL VIRGINIA.
I. Tagnon, W.J. Blot, N.E. Day, L.E. Morris, B.B. Peace
and J.F. Fraumeni Jr.

A case-control study, undertaken to clarify reasons for a
higher incidence of mesothelioma discovered among white
males in coastal Tidewater, Virginia, linked the high
rates to employment in area shipyards. The relative
risk (RR) of mesothelioma was 18.1 for career shipyard
workers who began employment before 1950 and were
reported to handle asbestos (95 percent confidence
limits = 8.1-48.4). The RR's were 16.4 for those who
worked only temporarily, most during World War II, and
were reportedly exposed to asbestos (95 per cent
confidence limits = 5.7-62.8), and 10.3 for career shipyard workers who began employment prior to 1950, and who
were not reported to handle asbestos (95 percent
confidence limits = 5.9-31.5). The risk of mesothelioma
was inversely associated with the amount of cigarettes
smoked, a trend that may be related to the powerful
competing risks for fatal diseases due to the interactions of smoking and asbestos exposure.

Environmental Epidemiology Branch, National Cancer
Institute, Bethesda, MD. 20205, U.S.A.
* Present address : Institut Médico-Social de la Province
de Brabant, rue de l'Hôpital, 35, 1000 Brussels, Belgium.

183

SURFACE MARKERS IN THREE CASES OF HAIRY CELL LEUKEMIA.
N.Tubiana, M.Derre, Y.Carcassonne

Hairy cell leukemia (HCL) has been an established clinicopath
ological & cytological entity for some 20 years but the
origin of the hairy cells is the subject of extensive de-
bate. Mononuclear cells of three patients with HCL were
examined for features suggestive of either a lymphocytic
or a monocytic origin. Suspensions of hairy cells were prepared by ficoll-hypaque centrifugation of heparinized peripheral blood or splenic cell suspensions.
-The three cell populations had low numbers of sheep erythrocyte rosettes (5-10%). After examination of cytocen-
trifuge E rosette preparations, only one preparation showed that rosetting cells were hairy cells. The results obtained with an anti-T cell serum were closely correlated
with the number of E rosettes.
-The three cell populations were negative for the C3 re-
ceptor(EAC).
-The cells were examined for surface immunoglobin (Ig)
after in vitro incubation which allows the dissociation
of serum-derived Ig adherent to FC receptor. Membrane
staining with fluorescein labelled monospecific antisera
against various Ig classes was negative in one subject; in
the two others the staining suggested the presence of multiple classes of Ig but staining was observed for three
heavy chains μ δ α in the first two, heavy chains μ γ in the
third, and for one light chain λ in the two cases. The aspect of this fluorescence was particular showing an aspect
of "capping".
-Methanol fixed cells were examined in order to detect intracellular immunoglobulins . The three preparations were
negative compared   to a control plasma cell preparation.
-The cell had minimal ability to phagocyte latex particles
These three cases confirm the diversity of the origin of
hairy cells.

Institut J.Paoli-I.Calmettes, Service d'Hématologie,
232 Bd Ste Marguerite, 13273 Marseille Cedex 2, France

184

IS ANDROGEN BINDING IN NORMAL AND PATHOLOGICAL LYMPHOCYTES
A "RECEPTOR"? N.Tubiana, P.M.Martin, P.H.Rolland,
Y.Carcassonne
The effects of androgens on lymphoid systems have been
described. In particular, the immuno-depressive effect
of testosterone has been demonstrated in vitro and in
vivo. In contrast, androgens are used as therapeutic agents
for some acute leukemic cells. The possible presence of
an androgen receptor in normal and pathological lymphoid
cells has been investigated, and the stability, specificity, cellular contents and nature and kinetic properties
of the steroid binding activity have been examined repeatedly in several collections of lymphocytes.
Androgen binding activity (ABA) in lymphocytes presents
some of the binding characteristics of a "typical" steroid
receptor : a) ABA could be inhibited by a 100-fold excess
of cold hormone, b) ^{3}H-R1881 shows specific binding as a
function of radioligand concentration and c) sucrose gradient analysis (SGA) evidence heavy centrifugation forms
for 1881. Furthermore, R-1881 is not metabolized by human
lymphocyte while dihydrotestosterone DHT is. However,
there are the following discrepancies to ascertain that
ABA is an androgen receptor : a) the specificity of DHT-
binding has been proved while that of R-1881 has not.
b) the dissociation constant Kd estimated for 1881 reveals low values (10^{-9}M) and c) DHT heavy centrifugation
forms were not observed by SGA. These discrepancies could
be attributed to (1) experimental conditions, since no
stabilisators were present in the incubation medium,
ATP content was not controlled and since the viability
of cells was determined only using dye-exclusion test.
(2) The fact that ABA was examined on lymphocytes + monocytes. In normal and pathological lymphocytes, androgen
binding content varied widely from subject to subject, but
also according to the number of cells present in the incubation medium.
Androgens bind to human lymphocytes, but the nature of this
binding activity remains to be determined.

Inst.J.Paoli-I.Calmettes,232 Bd Ste Marguerite,13009 Marseille

185

METHOTREXATE DIFFUSION IN CENTRAL NERVOUS SYSTEM (CNS).
N.Tubiana, S.Monjanel, D.Maraninchi, A.M.Imbert,J.A.Gastaut
J.P.Cano, Y.Carcassonne

The diffusion of MTX in CNS was studied in patients with lymphoblastic leukemia or lymphoma. The routes of administration studied included intrathecal injection (IT) and intravenous infusions. 1) Plasma MTX concentration after IT administration (15mg) in 10 subjects. The peak level of plasma MTX and its delay showed wide varations in C max (5 to 50 10^{-8}M) and in T max (2 to 40 H). This result was expected from analysis of pharmacokinectic data after IV ($50mg/m^2$) administration and from analysis of clinical toxicities and adverse reactions observed in some patients. The MTX plasmatic clearances after IT administration varied from 110 to 280 ml/mn and were quite similar to those obtained after IV bolus in the same subject. 2) The kinetics of translocation across the "blood brain barrier" in terms of entry into CSF (cerebral spinal fluid) after high dose infusions (8 or 36 H) was also studied in 6 patients. To prevent systemic toxicities,Citrovorum factor was started immediately at the end of the infusion at a dose of 12mg/m^2 every 6 H until the plasma MTX concentration was below 10^{-8}M. The MTX infusion dose was calculated to obtain a serum concentration plateau of 10^{-5}M during a 36 H infusion and a serum concentration of 10^{-4}M at the end of 8 H infusion. With 36 H MTX infusions, MTX level CSF peaked to 50 x 10^{-8}M. With 8 H MTX infusions, MTX level CSF peaked at 500 x 10^{-8}M. The CSF plasma MTX ratio was only about 1/20 at the peak in all these patients. The therapeutic concentration of about 10^{-6}M required for MTX to be effective in CNS was achieved during 8 H infusion without any neurotoxicity. These observations suggest that IV MTX can be as effective as IT MTX if given in a high enough dose and this systemic therapy had the advantage of providing consistent drug concentrations throughout the CSF axis.

Institut J.Paoli-I.Calmettes, Service d'Hématologie, 232 Bd Ste Marguerite, 13273 Marseille Cedex 2, France

186

LOW NATURAL-KILLER (NK) CELL ACTIVITY IN PATIENTS WITH MALIGNANT LYMPHOMA OR WITH A HIGH RISK FOR LYMPHOID TUMORS. T. Tursz, M.C. Dokhelar, M. Lipinski and J.L. Amiel.

Natural killer (NK) cell activity against K562 target cells was found to be decreased (mean value 27.5 %) in peripheral blood lymphocytes from 59 untreated patients with malignant lymphoma when compared to 112 healthy subjects (46.3 %) and to 75 cancer patients with non-lymphoïd tumors (43.7 %) (p<0.001). Low NK activity was also demonstrated in immunodepressed patients who have a known high risk of lymphoïd malignancies. This group included renal transplant recipients on immunosuppressive therapy and primary immunodeficiencies(ID) like Wiskott-Aldrich syndrome, ataxia-telangiectasia, severe combined ID, common variable ID and Chediak-Higashi syndrome. A role for NK cells in the immune surveillance against lymphoïd neoplasias is suggested.

Institut Gustave Roussy, 94800 Villejuif, France.

187

NATURAL KILLER ACTIVITY OF LYMPHOCYTES FROM CARCINOMATOUS PLEURAL EFFUSIONS OF CANCER PATIENTS
Atsushi Uchida and Michael Micksche

Lymphocytes and tumor cells were isolated from carcinomatous pleural effusions of patients with lung cancer by centrifugation on a discontinuous Ficoll-Hypaque gradient. Pleural effusion lymphocytes showed a higher percentage of sheep erythrocyte rosetting cells. NK activity was measured in a 4 hr 51-Cr release assay with human cultured cell lines (K562 etc.).PEL showed markedly low or no significant NK activity against highly sensitive K562 cells. NK activity of PEL was always lower than that of peripheral blood lymphocytes (PBL) of the same patients,which was lower compared to normal donors. When PEL were mixed with normal or cancer PBL and incubated for 24 hrs, significant suppression of NK activity of PBL was observed in 15 out of 20 PEL tested.Suppressor cells were found to be monocytes (80 % of the cases) and nylon wool nonadherent cells (20 %). When PEL were passed through a Sephadex G-10 column and cultured for 24 hrs, NK activity of PEL was significantly increased. Interferon and OK-432, a streptococcal preparation,augmented the NK activity of PEL. Purified tumor cells in pleural effusions were resistent to NK lysis and did not inhibit lysis of K562 cells in competition assay. Proliferative responses to PHA or ConA of PEL was higher compared to PBL of the same patients. Pleural effusion supernatant did not inhibit NK activity. The results suggest that carcinomatous pleural effusions contain potentially reactive NK cells, but these cells cannot mediate their lytic function because of the presence of suppressor cells.
Institute for Cancer Research, Univ. of Vienna, Austria

188

PHASE I STUDY OF 2-FORMYLPYRIDINE THIOSEMICARBAZONE ZINC SULPHATE(NSC294721)(PICAZONE).
J.Vanderlinden, R.De Jager, G.Atassi.

Picazone,a zinc chelate of 2-Formylpyridine thiosemicarbazone is a new chemotherapeutic agent with anti-tumor activity against P388 and L1210 leukemias including L1210 inoculated intracerebrally and inhibition of the formation of lung metastases in Lewis lung tumor. Picazone inhibits DNA synthesis by inhibiting ribonucleoside diphosphate reductase. Picazone in 250ml D5W was administered IV. over 30min. daily x5 every 21-28 days, escalating doses in the absence of toxicity. Fourteen patients with advanced solid tumors resistant to conventional therapy: head and neck(12),cervix(1),lung(1) received 27 courses.The daily dose was escalated as follows: 4, 8,12,20,32,50,130,210,250,340mg/m^2. The maximum tolerated daily dose was 340mg/m^2. Dose limiting toxicity was neurological. CNS toxicity consisting of confusion,disorientation,extrapyramidal signs,seizures and coma(1p) was reversible and dose-dependent between 210 and 340mg/m^2. No toxicity was seen below 130mg/m^2. Hematologic toxicity:hemoglobin drop > 1.5g%,leukopenia and thrombocytopenia occurred at 250(1p) and 340mg/m^2 (1p) with WBC nadirs of 1700 and 1600/mm^3 and platelet nadirs of 75000 and 120000/mm^3. Counts recovered by day 21. No definite proof of hemolysis was found.Black urine due to chelated iron probably mobilised from iron stores was seen at doses 130-340mg/m^2.No renal or hepatic toxicities were encountered.Nausea and/or vomiting occurred in one half of the patients. Transient minor anti-tumor effects were seen in 3 patients with head and neck tumors.The severe CNS toxicity makes this drug a poor candidate for phase II studies.
Institut J.Bordet - Brussels - BELGIUM.

48

189

INCREASED SENSITIVITY OF PERIPHERAL BLOOD LYMPHOCYTES FROM PATIENTS WITH HODGKIN'S DISEASE (HD) TO CONCANAVALIN A (ConA)-INDUCED SUPPRESSOR CELLS. C.P.Vanhaelen,R.I.Fisher.

We have established a method that reproducibly assays the response of peripheral blood lymphocytes to ConA-induced suppressor cells; using these techniques we have demonstrated that T cells from patients with active HD have increased sensitivity to the ConA-induced suppressor cell. Lymphocytes were incubated in culture media in the presence or absence of ConA, 50ug/ml for 48h, treated with mitomycinC, and their regulatory activity on the proliferation of fresh, allogeneic lymphocytes in response to a suboptimal (10ug/ml) dose of ConA was measured. The final cultures containing 10^5 fresh cells and 10^5 allogeneic regulator cells were incubated together for 48h, pulsed with tritiated thymidine, and harvested 24h later. The % suppression caused by ConA activated cells was calculated by the formula $100(NA - CA)/NA$ where NA represents the dpm of cultures containing non-activated regulator cells and CA represents cultures containing ConA-activated regulator cells. ConA-induced suppressor cells from 20 different normals suppressed normal allogeneic lymphocytes $38.7\pm3.0\%$. Lymphocytes from 12 patients with active HD suppressed allogeneic normal lymphocytes similarly ($36.7\pm3.1\%$). However, ConA-induced suppressor cells from normals caused significantly greater suppression of proliferation by lymphocytes from patients with HD ($57\pm4.9\%$, p<.001). This difference was not caused by the lower proliferation of Hodgkin's cells in response to ConA since identical results were obtained when normals with low ConA-induced proliferation were selected for comparison. Thus, although the ability to induce ConA-suppressor cells from peripheral blood of patients with HD is normal, patients with HD have increased sensitivity to suppression by ConA-induced regulator cells. Increased sensitivity to T cell regulation may explain some of the T cell deficits observed in patients with HD.

Medicine Branch, National Cancer Institute, Bethesda, MD, 20205, U.S.A.

190

CHANGES IN THE CELL MEMBRANE GLYCOPEPTIDES OF HUMAN LEUKAEMIC HAIRY CELLS. M.E. Van Rymenant, G.A.J.M. van der Hofstad, F.P. De Leeuw and J. Jansen.
Hairy-cell leukaemia (HCL) is an uncommon type of leukaemia. Its most striking morphological feature is the presence of many large microvilli at the surface of the leukaemic hairy cell. Since it has been established that the cell-surface glycoproteins of animal cells show changes upon malignant transformation (see Warren et al, Biochim. Biophys. Acta 516, 97-127, 1978) we compared the cell-surface glycopeptides of hairy cells with those of normal lymphocytes. The methods used were modified from Van Beek et al (Leukemia Res. 2, 163-171, 1978). Isolated cells were incubated in the presence of ^{3}H- or ^{14}C-fucose for hairy cells and control lymphocytes, respectively, and trypsinized afterwards. The trypsinates of ^{3}H-labeled HC and ^{14}C-labeled control lymphocytes were mixed and digested further with pronase (PRO). Part of the sample was treated with neuraminidase (NEU). The samples were fractionated on a Sephadex G50/Biogel P-10 column. ^{3}H- and ^{14}C-radioactivities of the fractions were determined. After PRO-digestion the HC glycopeptides of all 6 HCL-patients studied (3 obtained from peripheral blood cells and 3 from spleen cells obtained after splenectomy) show a reproducible shift to higher molecular weight (MW). Moreover the relative amount of the high MW glycopeptides is enhanced. In contrast to other types of leukaemia we have studied so far, this shift is not abolished upon NEU-treatment, but an increase of the shift is found. NEU is an enzyme which removes specifically the terminal sialic acid residues from the glycopeptides. After mild acid hydrolysis, which chemically splits off sialic acid residues, no differences in elution patterns remain. This supports the hypothesis that two kinds of sialic acid residues could exist in the fractionated glycopeptides : sialic acid residues free to react with neuraminidase and hidden sialic acid residues.

Laboratory of Medical Cancerology and Clinical Investigation, Cancer Center, Faculty of Medecine, Vrije Universiteit Brussel, Laarbeeklaan 103/E, 1090 Brussels (Belgium).

191

LEVAMISOLE IN COLORECTAL CANCER . H.Verhaegen, J.De Cree, W.De Cock, M.L.Verhaegen-Declercq

Sixty patients with operable colorectal cancer have been followed-up for at least five years after surgery.
Two groups of patients (each including 30 cases) were formed in such a way that they were well comparable for age, sex and Dukes' classification. Levamisole was started after surgery in one group whereas no further treatment was given to the control group.
When recurrent metastatic disease occurred, cytostatic treatment was started.
For the total population studied, the mortality was significantly lower in the Levamisole treated group.
Our data show that the benefit was most obvious in the patients with more advanced disease, i.e. Dukes B2 and C, Broders' classes III and IV.
A higher mortality was found in the patients from the control group when their pretreatment absolute lymphocyte counts were lower than the median value.
In the Levamisole treated group a significant increase in survival was found in the patients with lower absolute numbers of lymphocytes as compared to the control group.

Jan Palfijnziekenhuis, Lange Bremstraat # 70, 2060 Merksem, Belgium

192

BETA SUBUNIT OF HUMAN CHORIONIC GONADOTROPHIN (HCG) AND ALPHA FETO PROTEIN (AFP) IN DIAGNOSIS AND TREATMENT OF TESTICULAR CANCERS. D. Vugrin, W. Whitmore, R. Golbey

Nanogram measurements of HCG and AFP provide indispensable aid in the staging and monitoring of patients with germ cell tumors as demonstrated in 215 patients. Serum tumor markers (STM) are relatively insensitive for recognition of minimal metastatic disease and incidence of abnormal STM rises with increasing extent of metastatic disease. In 60 patients with stage II disease STM after orchiectomy and before lymphadenectomy (RPLND) suggested metastases in 45% of patients. Patients with elevated STM after RPLND are classified as stage III. STM were elevated in 87% (90/103) of patients with stage III disease and had prognostic significance. Complete responses (CR) to chemotherapy alone were highest in patients with normal STM (92%). Patients with elevated AFP had lower CRs than those without it (34% vs. 61%). High levels of AFP or HCG (>1000 ng/ml) were associated with decreased CR rates compared to lower levels (16% vs. 63%). 87% of patients with choriocarcinoma elements in the primary tumor had elevated HCG. 92% of patients with endodermal sinus elements in the primary tumor had elevated AFP. In a study of an additional 52 patients we found that those with serum HCG over 1000 ng/ml are at an increased risk for brain metastasis. Concomitant measurement of HCG in CSF and serum of patients with suspected CNS metastasis was useful in diagnosis and monitoring treatment. In conclusion, tumor markers are important in prognosis and management of patients with germ cell cancers.

Memorial Sloan-Kettering Cancer Center, 1275 York Avenue, New York, New York 10021, USA

193

CIS PLATINUM (CDDP) IN ADJUVANT COMBINATION CHEMOTHERAPY
OF RESECTED STAGE II TESTIS CANCER. D. Vugrin,
W. Whitmore, R. Golbey.

40-50% (range 20-80%) of patients with nonseminomatous
germ cell tumors (NSGCT) stage II following retroperitoneal lymph node dissection (RPLND) will relapse.
Early experience with relatively nontoxic adjuvant
chemotherapy using vinblastine, actinomycin D, bleomycin
and chlorambucil demonstrated that more aggressive
treatment is needed for stage II-B (relapse 36%).
Therefore 51 stage II-B patients following RPLND received
adjuvant high dose CDDP (120 mg/m^2) in the same
combination chemotherapy (VAB-3 or VAB-6) used for stage
III disease (for 2 or 1 years, respectively). None of
these 51 patients recurred with median follow-ups of 2
years for VAB-3 and 1 year for VAB-6. This demonstrates
effectiveness of chemoprophylaxis after RPLND in
prevention of recurrences in stage II-B disease. In view
of potential toxicity of such adjuvant chemotherapy it is
applied only to those at significant risk of relapse.
Patients with stage II-A disease ($\leqslant$ 5 LN positive,
largest LN $\leqslant$ 2cm) have low risk for recurrence and
similar survivals can probably be achieved with close
follow-up after RPLND and aggressive chemotherapy only
for those who relapse. Patients with stage II-B,
especially if metastases are bulky and/or extranodal
extension has occurred, will benefit from adjuvant
chemotherapy. Optimal combination and duration of
treatment remain to be defined.

Memorial Sloan-Kettering Cancer Center, 1275 York Avenue,
New York, New York 10021, USA

194

HIGH EFFECTIVENESS OF CIS-PLATINUM (CDDP) IN COMBINATION
CHEMOTHERAPY OF STAGE III GERM CELL TUMORS (GCT)
D. Vugrin, W. Whitmore, R. Golbey.

Between 1974 and 1979, 224 patients with stage III and
unresectable stage II germ cell tumors were treated with
one of 4 CDDP combination chemotherapy protocols (VABs 2,
3,4, and 5) and resulted in development of current,
highly effective therapeutic regimen VAB-6. Following
conclusions were drawn from preceding studies:
1)induction containing high dose CDDP is the most
effective part of chemotherapy and with closer intervals
between inductions relapses were reduced; 2) bulky
metastases have decreased complete remission (CR) rates
to chemotherapy alone, but long term CR can be achieved
with resection of residual disease and additional
chemotherapy; 3) long term maintenance is not necessary;
4) initial chemotherapy should be the optimal regimen
as the majority of CR are achieved with initial
treatment and patients who fail prior chemotherapy fare
poorly. VAB-6 is given for 1 year and starts with 3
successive 4 day inductions given 3-4 weeks apart.
Induction is: Day 1 Cyclophosphamide 600 mg/m^2 IV,
Vinblastine (VLB) 4 mg/m^2 IV, Actinomycin D 1 mg/m^2 IV,
Bleomycin 30 mg IV; day 1-3 Bleo 20 mg/m^2/day x3 by
continuous 24 hr. infusion; day 4 CDDP 120 mg/m^2 IV. The
3rd induction omits Bleo. 1 month after 3rd induction
residual disease is resected. Patients who have adult
teratoma or no tumor in resected specimen are placed
on maintenance with Vlb 6 mg/m^2 IV and Act-D 1 mg/m^2 IV
Q 3 weeks. If resected specimen contains malignant
tissue an additional 2 inductions are given before
maintenance. 92% (23/25) of evaluable patients achieved
CR on VAB-6. 84% (21/23) CRs remain in CR. Myelosuppression is principal toxicity with 12% patients
requiring systemic antibiotics. VAB-6 protocol
demonstrates high efficacy of relative short course of
modern chemotherapy with very good tolerance.

Memorial Sloan-Kettering Cancer Center, New York, N.Y.

195

NONSPECIFIC CROSS-REACTING ANTIGEN IN NORMAL AND LEUKEMIC
MYELOID CELLS AND SERUM OF LEUKEMIC PATIENTS. B.Wahren,
G.Gahrton, S.Hammarström

Nonspecific cross-reacting antigen (NCA) could be demonstrated in myeloid cells from 20 nonleukemic persons, 16
patients with acute nonlymphoblastic leukemia and 8 patients with chronic myelocytic leukemia. Two independent
methods were used : immunofluorescence combined with micro-
fluorometry of single cells, and radioimmunoassay of lysates of bone marrow or separated cell fractions.
In both nonleukemic and leukemic cells, the NCA values
were high in neutrophils and low or non-detectable in
mononuclear cells. In the bone marrow, myelocytes and
metamyelocytes usually had higher individual NCA immunofluorescence values than did neutrophils. Myeloblasts and
erythroblasts had no detectable NCA. Bone marrow cells
cultured in vitro contained NCA. Carcinoembryonic antigen
was low or not detectable in all blood and bone marrow
cells.
Serum NCA was raised to a mean of 262 ng NCA per ml for
chronic myelocytic leukemia patients, compared to 51 ng/ml
for nonleukemic and 55 ng/ml for acute nonlymphoblastic
leukemia patients. The raised serum NCA was related to an
increased number of immature and mature myeloid cells in
the peripheral blood of leukemic patients and could reach
values over 500 ng/ml in untreated subjects.

Statens, Bakteriologiska Laboratorium, 105 21 Stockholm,
Sweden

196

TYPING OF ALLOGENEIC MELANOMA LINES FOR MELANOMA VACCINIA
ONCOLYSATE TRIALS. M.K. Wallack, E. Leftheriotis,
J. Carcagne, P. Noël, C. Bailly, B.Fontanière, H. Cabril-
lat, S.Bertrand, A.Weissbrod, K.Gronneberg, J.F.Doré and
M.Mayer.

12 patients with recurrent Stage II malignant melanoma
have been treated in a phase I trial with repeated intradermal injections of vaccinia viral oncolysates prepared from allogeneic melanoma lines. 5/12 patients
showed lack of progression of disease while receiving
therapy and lived longer than the expected survival of
6 months.

Since the survival data points to the possibility of
immunotherapy with allogeneic melanoma lines, characterization of these lines for tumorigenicity and antigenicity becomes quite important. The following studies are
performed on each melanoma line to establish the quality of the preparation : (1) cytology (2) electronmicros-
copy (3) karyotyping (4) growth in nude mice and
(5) characterization of melanoma antigens on the melanoma cells and in the melanoma oncolysates with wistar
melanoma monoclonal antibody.

Approximately 31 melanoma lines have been established
and tested. The above tests verify the antigenicity and
tumorigenicity of these lines so that they can be used
for the production of melanoma vaccinia oncolysates for
human trials.

Centre Léon Bérard, 28 rue Laënnec 69373 Lyon Cedex 2
and Institut Mérieux, Marcy 1'Etoile 69260 Charbonnières
Les Bains - France.

50

197

AN IMMUNOLOGIC ASSESSMENT IN PATIENTS WITH UTERINE CERVIX CARCINOMA.

P.Wattré, F.Santoro, A.Capron, J.Bonneterre, R.Beuscart, MC.Vie, P.Cappelaere, A.Demaille

Immunologic parameters have been studied before treatment in 111 patients (pts) with intraepithelial epithelioma (12 pts:group I),invasive epithelioma stage I or II(57 pts:group II) and stage III or IV(42 pts:group III).With various concentrations of mitogens,the lymphoblastogenesis was significantly reduced in group III vs group II patients with phytohemagglutinin (PHA)(6,12,25 µg/100 µl)and Concanavalin A(ConA)(6,12,25,50 µg/100µl) and in group II vs group I patients with pokeweed mitogen (PWM)(12,25, 50 µg/100ul).B lymphocytes (S.Ig immunofluorescence) and T lymphocytes (T rosettes) number and percentage were unchanged whatever the stage. The mean values of carcinoembryonic antigen (CEA) and the rate of pathologic values (>10ng/ml) were elevated in group III patients. 41 % of all patients had circulating immune complexes(C.I.C.) (≭ C1q binding) whatever the stage. The mean values of complement factors CH50,C1q,C3a and C1 inhibitor were unchanged but those of C3c and C4 were significantly elevated in group III patients. Immuno-globulin A was elevated in group III patients but not immunoglobulin G and M. Anti ADN auto-antibodies (hemagglutination and immunofluorescence) were never found. 45 % of patients had positive skin test with tuberculin. Multivariate analysis found some associations between clinical and immunological parameters : age of patients, complement factors and C.I.C. were associated ; lymphoblastogenesis with PHA and ConA were closely correlated too. Linear regression tests demonstrated a relationship between PHA lymphoblastogenesis and positive tuberculin skin test and between C.I.C and CEA, IgA, IgM, C1q and C3a. Immunologic parameters in our patients show a significant decrease of lymphoblastogenesis, early with PWM.Moreover,C3c, C4, IgA and CEA are elevated in patients with advanced disease Centre O. LAMBRET,BP 307, rue F.Combemale,59020 LILLE CEDEX, FRANCE

198

A MONOCLONAL ANTIBODY DEFINING A BURKITT LYMPHOMA ASSOCIATED ANTIGEN. J. Wiels[1], M. Fellous[2] and T. Tursz[1].

We have produced monoclonal antibodies by the technique of cell fusion, using the myeloma line SP2OAg14 and Lewis rat splenocytes sensitized in vivo with Daudi cells (Burkitt derived cell line expressing neither HLA-A,B and C molecules nor β-2 microglobulin). After cell fusion selection and cloning of hybrid cells, hybridoma supernatants were tested in C' - dependent cytotoxicity, indirect immunofluorescence and radioactive binding assays against cells from a panel of lymphoïd cells of various origins. One hybridoma supernatant (38.13) contained IgM antibodies reacting with cells from Burkitt lymphoma derived lines, regardless of whether or not they contained the EBV genome. No reactivity was observed with T cell lines or B cell lines originated from in vitro EBV infected normal B lymphocytes. 38.13 did not react with normal B cells and with malignant cells from patients with various leukemias or non- Burkitt lymphomas. The monoclonal antibody 38.13 thus appeared to recognize a Burkitt lymphoma associated antigen.

1. Institut Gustave Roussy, 94800 Villejuif, France.
2. Hôpital Saint-Louis, Paris, France.

199

ANTIEMETICS FOR PATIENTS TREATED WITH ANTITUMOUR CHEMOTHERAPY. C.J. Williams, R. de Pemberton, J.M.A. Whitehouse

The antiemetic effects of metoclopramide and cyclizine were studied in a group of patients receiving antitumour chemotherapy. Each patient received the following antiemetic regimes in random sequence a) Placebo; b) Cyclizine; c) metoclopramide and d) cyclizine and metoclopromide. All drugs were given double-blind using a double dummy technique. The anti-emetic treatment was started 3 hours before the antitumour chemotherapy and continued in a 6 hour oral schedule for 24 hours.

The degree of nausea and vomiting and the side effects of the antiemetic treatment were assessed by a self-administered questionaire using a linear analogue scale. No significant reduction in nausea and vomiting were seen with these regimes though Nabilone and metoclopramide appeared to be active in a pilot study. The trial design used is simple and statistically efficient and will be discussed further.

CRC Medical Oncology Unit, Southampton, England.

200

CHEMOTHERAPY OF ADVANCED OVARIAN CARCINOMA. RESULTS OF A MULTIPLE CHEMOTHERAPY COMBINATION PROTOCOL. J.P.Wolff, M.George

29 cases of advanced ovarian carcinomas (stage III-IV) were treated with a sophisticated combination of chemotherapy : Adriamycin, VM 26, Endoxan, 5 FU, Cytembena, Cis-platinum. The side-effects were low, except for Cytembena which seems to be responsible for renal complications and was stopped.
Out of 29 cases, 5 complete remissions and 3 over 50 percent remissions were observed ; all are longer than 6 months; all but one were verified by second-look operation. If patients without previous treatment only are taken into consideration, the number of remissions is 8/23 (instead of 8/29).

Service de Gynécologie, Institut Gustave-Roussy, Hautes Bruyères, Rue Camille Desmoulins, 94800 Villejuif, France

201

DIRECT HUMAN IN VIVO EFFECT OF MALIGNANT TUMOR UPON IM-
MUNITY IN BREAST CANCER PATIENTS.J .Wybran and
W . Matthelem.

In nine patients with breast cancer, the tumor was exci-
sed and in a dynamic in vivo system, humoral and cellular non specific immunity were studied in the main af-
ferent blood supply to the tumor as well as in the main
efferent blood return from the tumor.This system allows
thus to directly investigate the immunological modifications due to the tumor itself. No changes were observed in the levels of total complement, third and
fourth factors of complement , IgA and IgM. In contrast,
IgG levels increased in the efferent blood of 4 patients (average 100 mg %). There were no changes in the
percentages of EAC rosettes . The efferent blood showed
an increase in the percentages of total T rosettes in
3 patients and a decrease in 3 other patients. The
major change in the efferent blood was observed using
the active T rosette test : 8 patients showed a decrease in their percentage of active T rosettes. No changes in the spontaneous thymidine incorporation or the
lymphocyte response to phytohemagglutinin were observed.

In conclusion it appears that the blood passage through
the tumor produces an increase in IgG levels and a decrease in active T rosettes. This latter finding suggests that the non specific cellular immunodefi-
ciency seen in cancer patients is explained at least
partly by the presence of the tumor rather than by a
primary defect in cell mediated immunity.

Saint Pierre and Erasme Hospital, Departments of
Immunology and Hematology and Bordet Tumor Institute,
Department of Surgery,Free University of Brussels,
1000 Brussels , Belgium.

202

NPT 15392, A NEW SYNTHETIC IMMUNOMODULATORY AGENT : HU-
MAN PRECLINICAL AND CLINICAL RESULTS. J. Wybran and
J. Schmerber

NPT 15392 , a new synthetic drug, was investigated in
various human assays both in vitro and in vivo for
its potential immunological properties. NPT 15392 was
studied for its action upon various rosette assays according the following procedure : peripheral blood was
first incubated with various concentrations of the
drug (from 0.0001 µg/ml to 10 µg/ml) and then tested in the rosette systems . It was found that NPT 15392
significantly increased the percentages of active T
rosettes already at a concentration of 0.001 µg/ml
(p < 0.02 compared to controls) and up to 10 µg/ml
(p < 0.0001) . NPT 15392 did not modify the percentage of total T rosettes, human autologous T rosettes, or
EAC rosettes . In vivo,four cancer patients re- .
ceived orally a single dose of 0.7 mg. All four cancer
patients showed a significant increase and normalisa-
-tion in the percentages of blood active T rosettes,
autologous T rosettes and total T rosettes . This
effect was already observed at 24 hours and lasted between 24 and 48 hours. Three cancer patients received an oral dose of 0.4 mg and showed an increase
and normalisation of active T rosettes on day 2 or
day 3. In conclusion , NPT 15392 has shown to be,
both in vitro and in vivo, a drug with T cell mo-
dulatory effect. In cancer patients , it completely
and rapidly restores non specific cellular immunity.

Saint-Pierre and Erasme Hospital, Departments of Immunology and Hematology, Free University of Brussels,
1000 Brussels, Belgium.

203

VALUE OF ECHOCARDIOGRAPHY IN CHILDREN TREATED BY ADRIAMY-
CIN : A PROSPECTIVE STUDY IN 52 PATIENTS. J.M.Zucker,
L.Fermont, B.Asselain, E.Margulis, N.Lemercier

From July 1978 to June 1980, 52 patients aged 1 to 15
years were investigated by 2 to 7 serial M-mode, and oc-
casionally cross-sectional, echocardiograms. There were
35 solid tumors and 17 lymphomas receiving a multidrug
treatment including adriamycin.
The left ventricular function was assessed by shortening
fraction (SF), left pre-ejection period to ejection time
ratio (LPEP/ET), isovolumetric contraction time (ICT),ve-
locity of circumferential fiber shortening (VLF) and left
ventricular ejection fraction (EF). The results were compared with the clinical, radiological and electrocardio-
graphical data.
Reliability of each of the five selected parameters was
asserted by a significant correlation between their changes and the cumulative dose of adriamycin (p=0.05 to 0.01).
Impairment of the myocardial function increased progressively up to a 300 mg/m^2 dose, then dramatically between
350 to 450 mg/m^2. High doses of cyclophosphamide and methotrexate as well as radiotherapy on the chest were shown
to be aggravating factors : in 4 patients the drug had to
be postponed after 180 to 420 mg/m^2, and 3 others displayed severe cardiomyopathy before reaching 450 mg/m^2.
In view of these results, the significance of echocardio-
graphic changes in a given patient and the subsequent
therapeutic deductions are questioned:
- cardiotoxicity may occur for lower doses than it is
usually claimed.
- children receiving adriamycin should be monitored by
serial echocardiograms, tentatively prior to therapy, at
180 mg/m^2, and before each further dose.
- if all parameters deteriorate progressively, withhold-
ing the drug or delaying its administration has to be
seriously discussed.

Institut Curie, 26 rue d'Ulm, 75231 PARIS Cedex 05,France

204

MULTIPLE BIOCHEMICAL MARKERS IN FOLLOW-UP OF OVARIAN
CANCER, W.G.Haije, E.H.Cooper, S.Haworth, J.Meerwaldt
& A.Roberts

In 31 patients treated for ovarian cancer and
followed for >2 years a battery of biochemical
markers were evaluated. They included: Phosphohexose
isomerase (PHI), C-reactive protein (CRP), α_1 Acid
Glycoprotein, Albumin (ALB), Pre-albumin (PAB),
Transferrin (TSF), β2-Microglubulin (β2-m), Sex
hormone binding globulin, Carcinoembryonic antigen
(CEA) and Placental-like Alkaline Phosphatase (PAP).

In 10 patients who had no evidence of disease during
follow-up, the markers stayed almost without
exception within normal limits with only minor
fluctuations. In some patients raised CEA was found.
Of 5 patients with tumours who responded favourably
to therapy, some markers were raised when tumour was
present (PAP 5x, PHI 2x, CRP 1x) and returned to
normal afterwards. CEA showed less consistent values.
The other markers had normal values.
16 patients did not respond to therapy: the tumours
tended to progress or there were recurrences. 12 of
them died during follow-up.
In this group of badly controlled patients, many
biochemical disturbances were found: PAP & CEA were
often raised, sometimes progressively; PHI & β2-m
values in many patients fluctuated above the normal
level. In most cases a significant drop in ALB values
(accompanied by declining PAB & TSF concentrations)
was seen together with a marked rise of CRP levels.

Longitudinal studies of some of these markers have
potential as an aid to contribute to the management
of patients with ovarian cancer.

Rotterdamsch Radio-Therapeutisch Instituut,
Rotterdam.

Recent Results in Cancer Research

Volume 72

Hairy Cell Leukemia

Editors: J.C. Cawley, G.F. Burns, F.G.J. Hayhoe

1980. 64 figs., 4 tab. IX, 123 pages
Cloth DM 56,–; approx. US $33.10
ISBN 3-540-09920-4

Contents: Introduction.– Clinical Aspects.– Pathology.– The Hairy Cell: Cytological Aspects.– The Hairy Cell: Immunological Aspects.– Other Haemic Cells.– Diagnosis.– Conclusion and Future Trends.– References.– Subject Index.

This monograph is the first comprehensive account of the various aspects of hairy cell leukaemia. Based on the author's own vast experience in the study and treatment of leukaemic disorders, it reflects the intense research activity the disease has attracted in the last 10 years.

The clinical aspects of hairy cell leukaemia are reviewed in detail following a brief introductory chapter. Subsequent sections deal with the pathology of the disease, the pathognomonic hairy cell, the involvement of other haemic cell types and differential diagnosis. Special attention is given to the often controversial cytological and immunological studies on the nature and origin of the hairy cell.

This unique work will be of interest to clinicians, laboratory haematologists and immunologists alike.

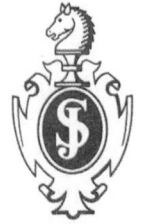

Springer-Verlag Berlin Heidelberg New York

Recent Results in Cancer Research   Volume 72

Hairy Cell Leukemia

Springer-Verlag Berlin Heidelberg New York